H is for HORSE

An easy guide to veterinary care for horses

Dr. Terrie Sizemore DVM

Library of Congress Control Number: 2017904336

First Edition 2017

Printed in the United States of America
A 2 Z Press LLC
PO Box 582
Deleon Springs, FL 32130
szemore3630@aol.com
bestlittlonlinebookstore.com
386-681-7402

ISBN: 978-0-9976407-6-2

Dedication

This book is dedicated in memory
of my beloved grandfather,
Alexander Balcziunas.

TABLE OF CONTENTS

PREFACE

I have been a busy veterinarian for many years and have had the unique experience of meeting people from many backgrounds in my varied practice.

I have observed that horse owners would like to learn, know, feel confident, and understand more about the care the horses they love and engage with every day benefit from.

It is my intent to create a book that simplifies technical medical information so horse owners and readers become informed without being overwhelmed. I hope to eliminate the frustration some owners face and encourage owners and readers to continue their quest for knowledge. I am convinced informed owners make better owners and will make better decisions for their horses.

It is also my hope that every owner and reader not only enjoys the basic and easy to understand information in this book but that, after reading it, they can, with confidence, seek great care for their horses.

This book is written to provide owners with basic general information regarding horse needs and care.

This work is not intended to be a substitute for veterinary care. No one can learn the professional discipline of being a veterinarian from a book. You, as the reader, will quickly realize many disorders overlap in signs and symptoms and there is caution to not overlook serious illness as much as not to mistake simple, uncomplicated disorders for more serious illness.

Please seek veterinary care for your pet as needed. Some situations encountered with your beloved pets require immediate attention.

Enjoy this book! Terrie Sizemore DVM

INTRODUCTION

Dogs and cats are close companions; however, every horse lover and owner knows that horses can also be close companions.

Every day in my chosen professions, I make technical medical information understandable to my clients and patients.

Horses have many roles in the lives of some people, however, most are companion animals to individuals and children. They are fun company for their owners as well as can make childhood a most memorable time.

I was a typical young girl who loved horses and wanted to spend my life with them. I have had the opportunity to ride and race and train and breed horses for many years. Each has its own distinct personality and added much enjoyment to my life as well as to owners I have come to know over the years. Keeping them healthy and with their owners and families is what I do every day.

"H is for Horse" provides basic knowledge for every horse owner. The subjects range from vaccines for major preventable diseases in horses to reasons for castrating, breeding horses, arthritis, dental care, emergency care, performing a physical exam, geriatric concerns, nutritional care for horses, poisonous plants and substances to horses, and a very brief chapter on behavioral issues.

Chapter 1

Picking the Perfect Horse for You

Horses are ..... .

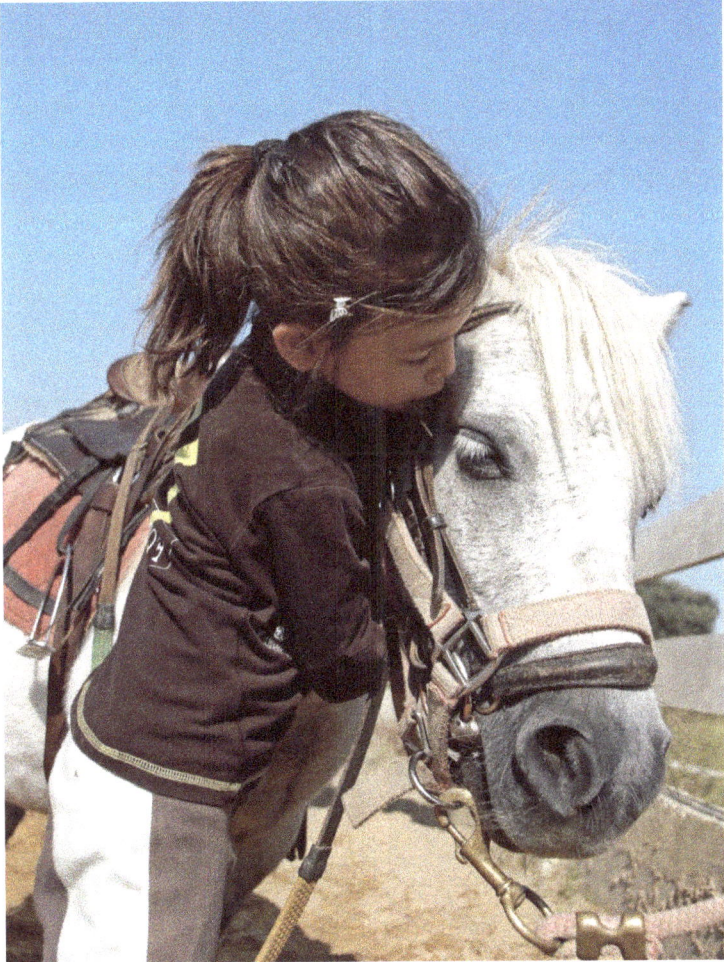

..... many girls' best friends!

Whether you decide you would like to…

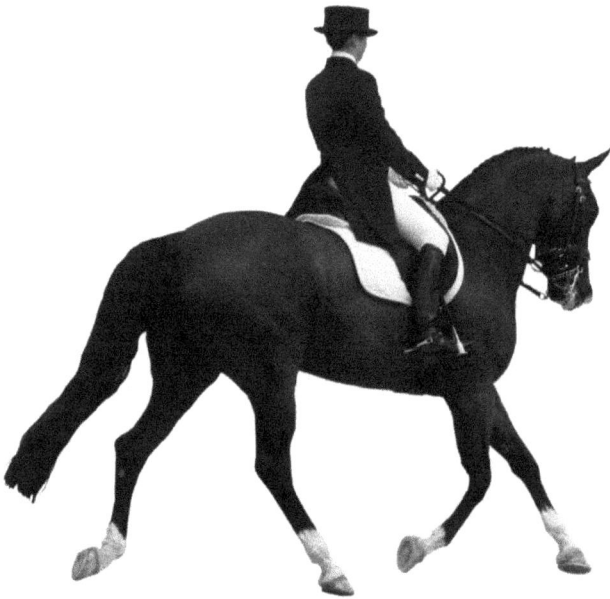

……ride English style…..
………like this dressage horse…..

.......or Western.....

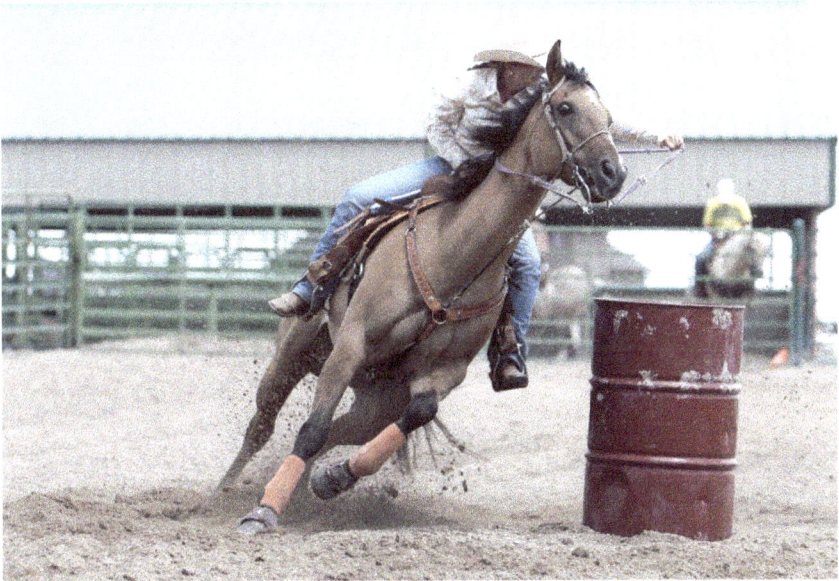

....like this barrel racing horse.....

....or you need your horse ...

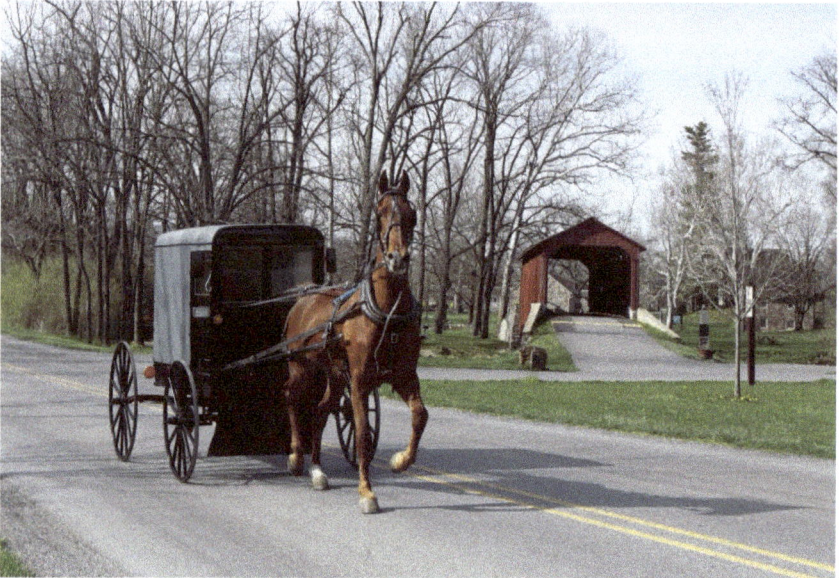

...for transportation.......

......have aspirations of being ....

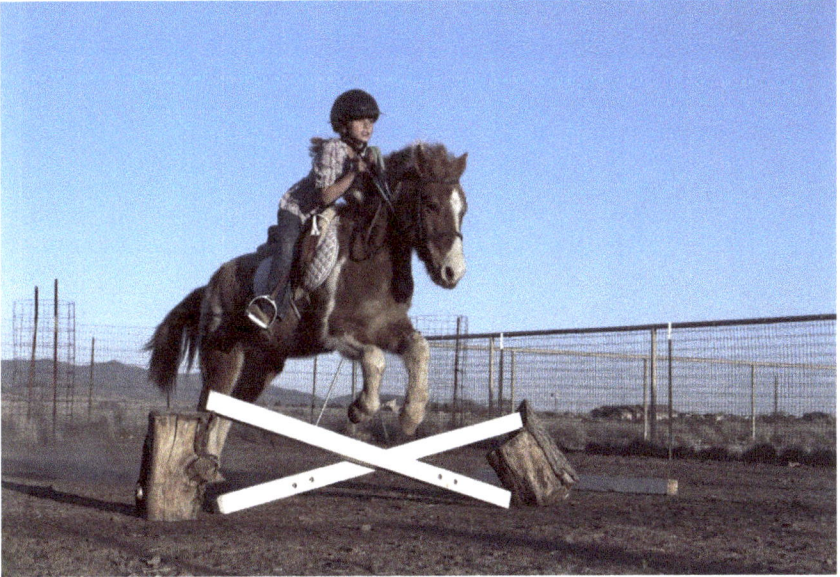

....a show jumper.....

......or want a horse.....

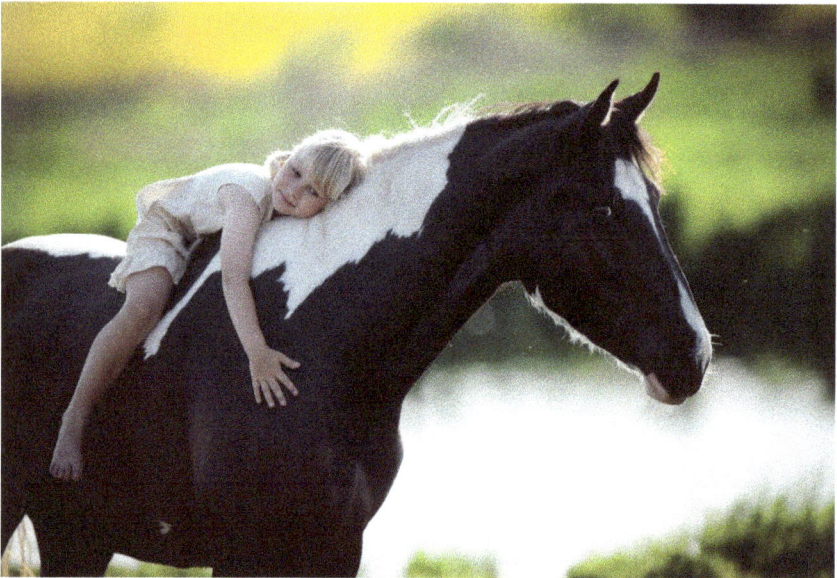

.... just for the pure pleasure......

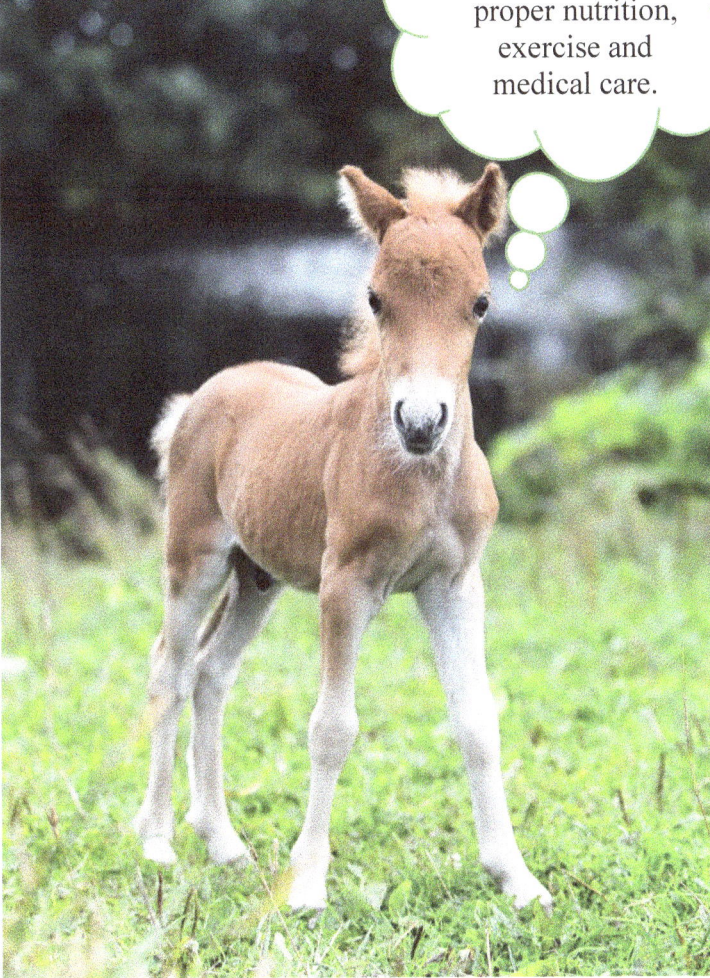

Just like the rest of the family, our horses need proper nutrition, exercise and medical care.

So, don't forget to pick a veterinarian for you and your horse.

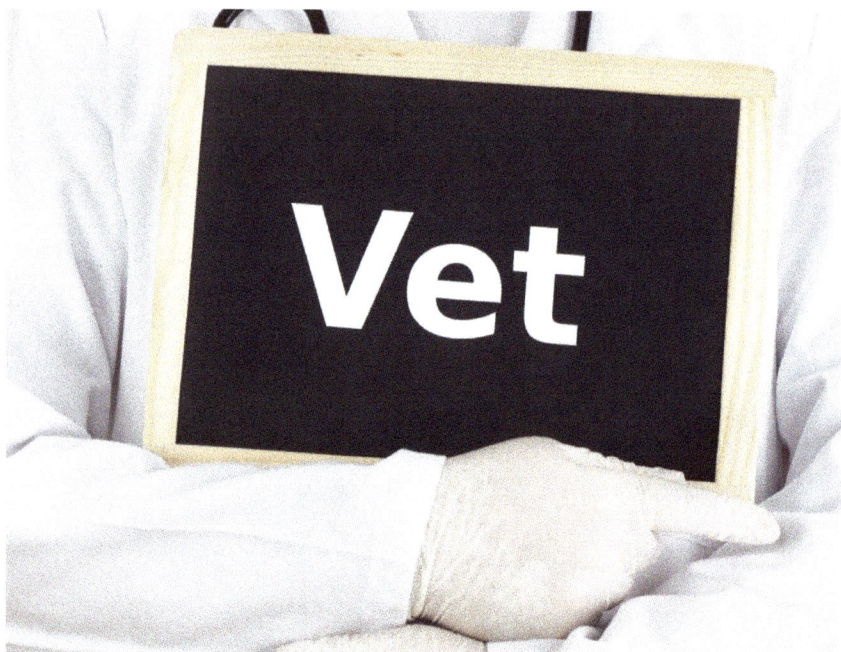

Veterinarians are committed to the best care for your horse and are certain you want to understand care recommendations so you as owners can make great choices for your furred (and sometimes not furred) friends.

PICKING A VETERINARIAN

WHAT TO CONSIDER WHEN CHOOSING YOUR PET'S DOCTOR

Some clinics provide
- general service
- some are exclusive or mixed for horses
- some service farm animals
- some are 'cats only'- don't pick them!
- some treat birds, fish, reptiles, and exotics but may also see horses

Other clinics have specialists for advanced care for:
- surgical needs
- skin diseases
- bone care
- eye/ear/neurological issues
- and other specialty concerns

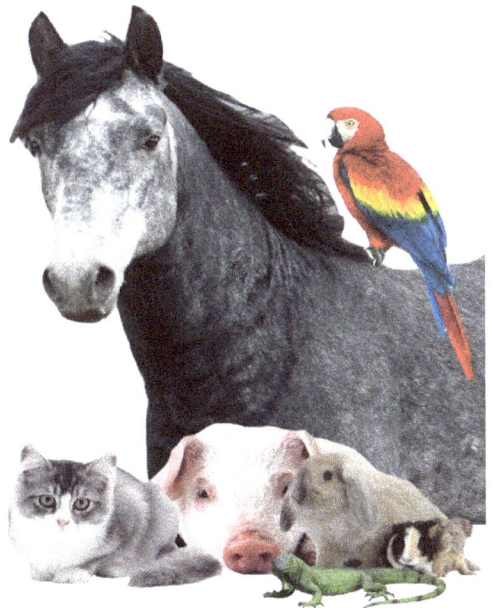

There are many great veterinarians to assist with your horse needs.

Now that we have welcomed our horses, some basic topics of pet care included here are:

1. vaccines
2. tick diseases
3. castrating horses
4. what to expect when your mare is expecting
5. dental care (teeth)
6. nutrition
7. lameness and arthritis
8. pet poisons
9. training and behavior
10. frequently recommended testing
11. emergency care for horses
12. care for senior horses
13. and more!

Chapter 2

Vaccines and Disease

Many years ago, scientists studied germs and disease. No one believed very small, microscopic 'things'—AKA germs—could enter a person's or pet's body and cause disease.

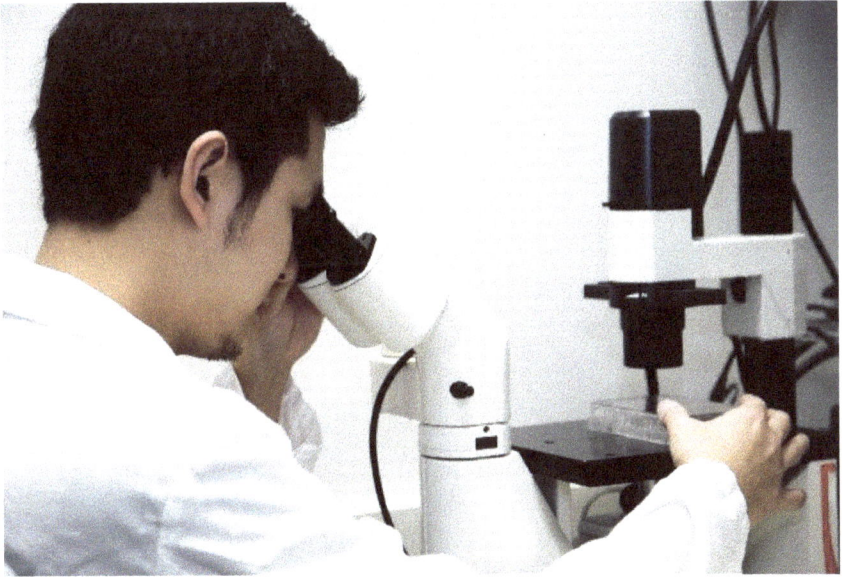

"GERMS" include:

- bacteria
- viruses
- fungi—which includes yeast and molds

THE MAJOR PREVENTABLE
DISEASES OF HORSES

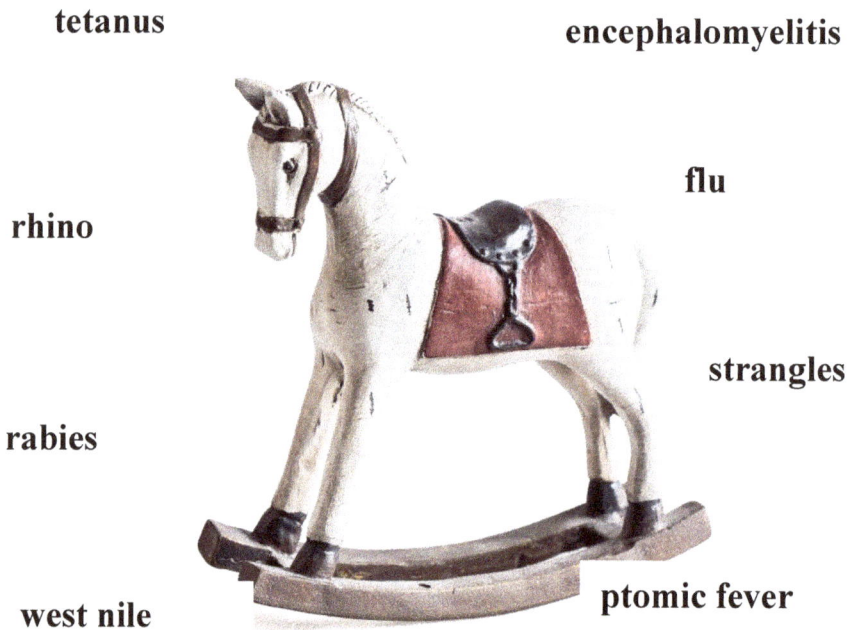

tetanus

encephalomyelitis

flu

rhino

strangles

rabies

west nile

ptomic fever

Today more is known about germs and disease. Microscopic organisms do indeed cause diseases that affect our horses.

TRANSMISSION OF GERMS

Horses encounter infectious organisms—GERMS—that cause all the following diseases by:

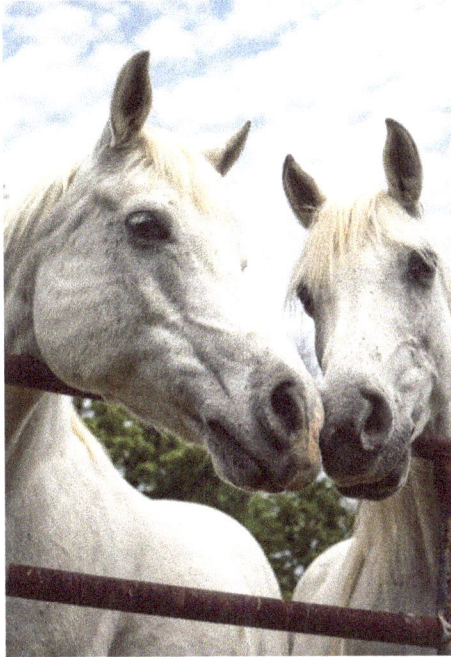

- touch—direct contact from horse to horse
- mother horses transferring disease to their babies – either through the placenta when pregnant, through milk when nursing, or direct contact after birth
- exposure to fecal material, (AKA poop)
- exposure to the saliva of infected horses
- wildlife—such as raccoons, skunks, coyotes, rodents, and more carry germs that cause disease
- fleas, mosquitoes and ticks
- exposure to water—puddles, lakes, and other waterways contaminated with disease-causing germs
- "fomites"—objects that carry germs: like boots, pants legs, feed tubs, tack, grooming equipment, and other physical objects

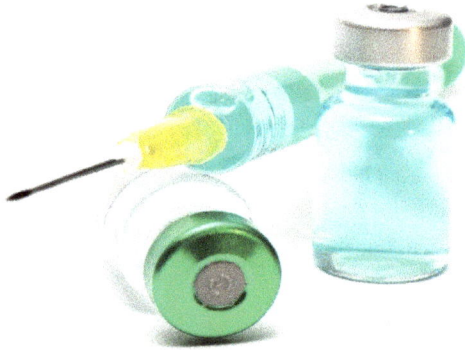

Scientists created vaccines to protect horses from disease.

When well horses are vaccinated, they make protective proteins called antibodies against the diseases they are vaccinated for. This protection allows them to fight infection if exposed to real germs.

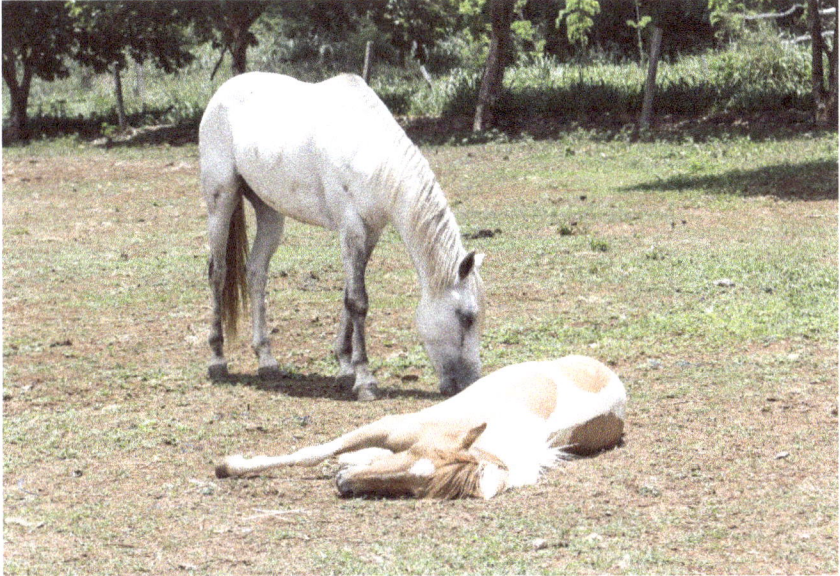

Goals when vaccinating are:

- horses will not become ill
- or, the illness will be less severe

THE VACCINE CONTROVERSY

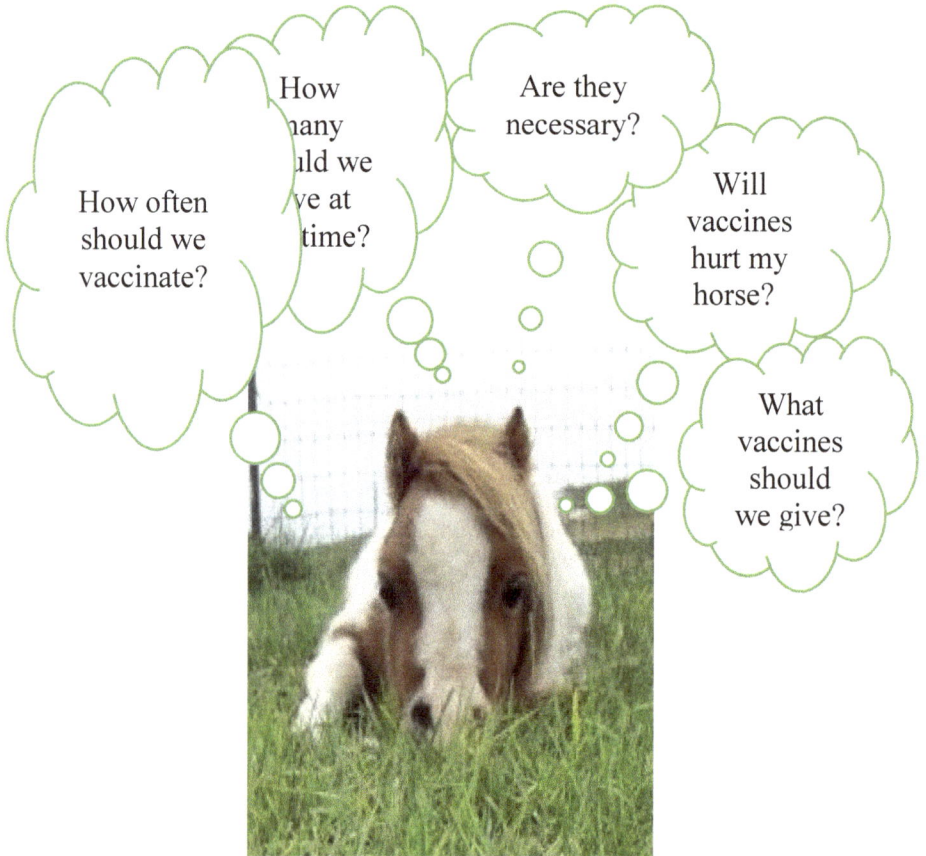

Despite the controversy over vaccinating, and while it is true there are minimal risks to vaccinating horses………

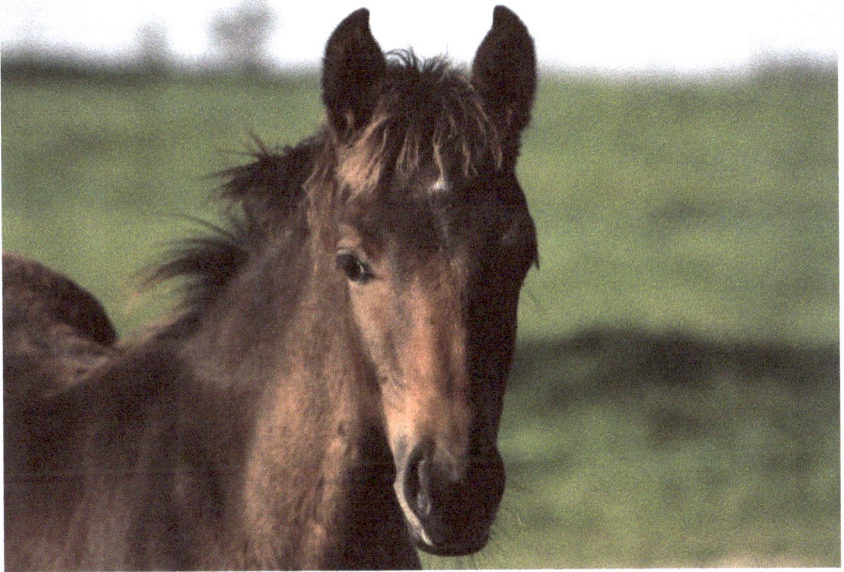

…..it is still the number one and best way to minimize or eliminate illness in our horses.

Vaccinating is not a method of treating illness or a cure for the diseases outlined in the pages to follow, but a means of *preventing* illness.

It has been proven that the risks of disease are far greater than the risks of vaccinating. For many of the diseases horses may encounter, some of the vaccines are essential for health- for example- tetanus.

Vaccine

A vaccine ~~ biological pr
improves immunity to a p
disease. A vaccine typic:
agent that resembles a
microorganism, and is
weakened or killed fc
or its toxins. The ag
body's immune sy
foreign,

When a horse is exposed to germs that cause disease, there is a delay in their creating the protective proteins (antibodies) needed to fight the infection.

While creating these antibodies, a horse can become very ill during this time and may be lost before they can fight the infection.

Also, infections may result in long-term negative effects.

In addition to preventing disease and loss of horses from disease, vaccinating lowers the cost of care of our horses. Diagnostic testing and treating horses that become ill is expensive and time-consuming, and it can be devastating for owners who love their pets.

Vaccines are available and recommended for:

- equine encephalomyelitis (sleeping sickness)
- equine influenza (flu)
- streptococcus equi (strangles)
- rhinopneumonitis/equine herpesvirus (EHV)
- west nile virus
- tetanus (lockjaw)
- rabies
- ptomic horse fever

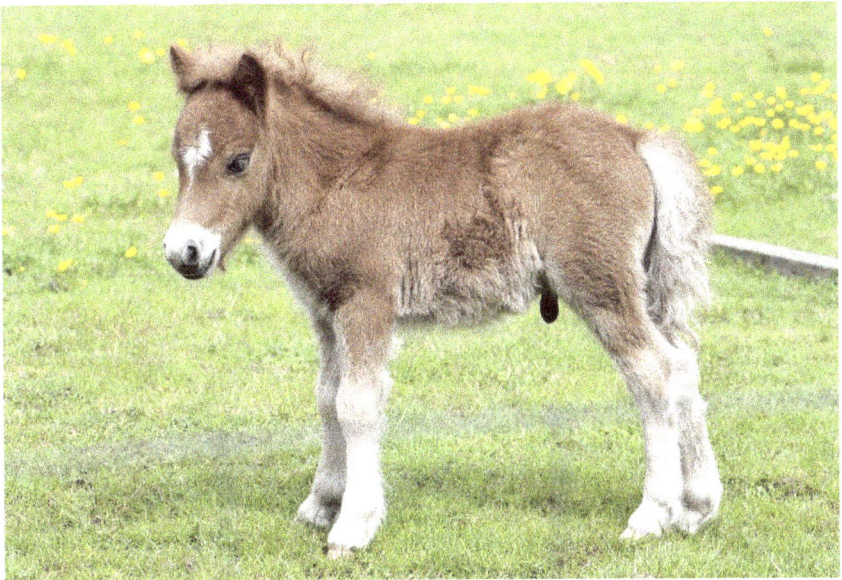

other diseases that may affect horses are:

- equine protozoal myeloencephalitis (EPM)
- equine infectious anemia virus (EIA)

… however, there is currently no vaccine for these diseases.

Equine Encephalomyelitis

Equine encephalomyelitis (en- seff - a- low- my- ell- eye- tis) – is also known as sleeping sickness. It is often a fatal disease that attacks the brain and spinal cord of infected horses.

Encephalomyelitis is caused by viruses in the family of equine encephalomyelitis viruses known as the *Togaviridae* family.

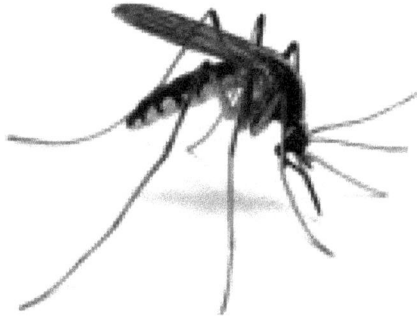

Encephalomyelitis is transmitted from horse to horse by mosquitoes.

Three common strains are Eastern (EEE), Western (WEE), and Venezuelan (VEE) encephalomyelitis. This is a disease humans can acquire as well as horses, burros, donkeys, and zebra.

Eastern (EEE) is the deadliest, killing 75-100% of infected horses.

Signs of encephalomyelitis include:

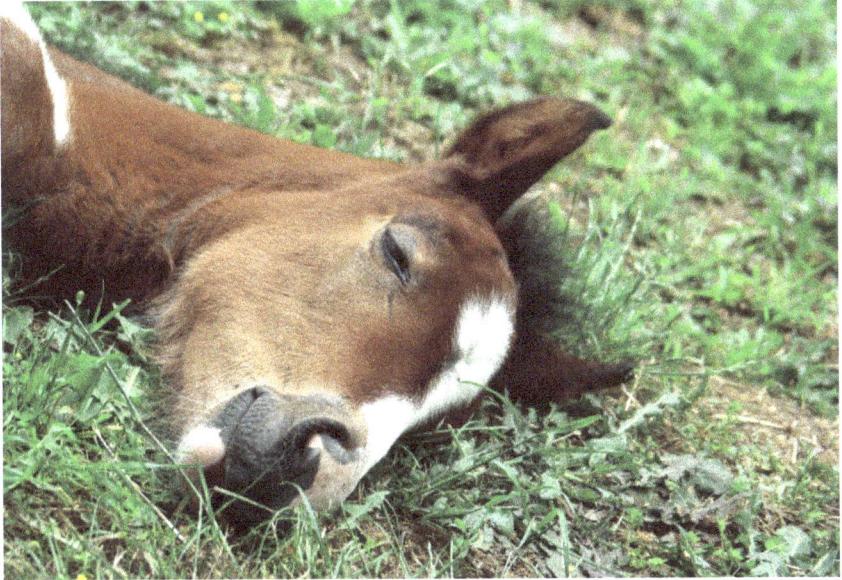

- depression
- loss of appetite
- fever
- which is sometimes followed by a period where a horse may appear excited or
- blind- walking into objects
- nervous
- and uncoordinated and
- have muscle tremors
- and eventually, the horse may become completely paralyzed

Surviving horses may suffer permanent damage.
.

Western (WEE) is more common and somewhat less devastating. Both EEE and WEE can occur throughout the U.S., and horses should be vaccinated for both.

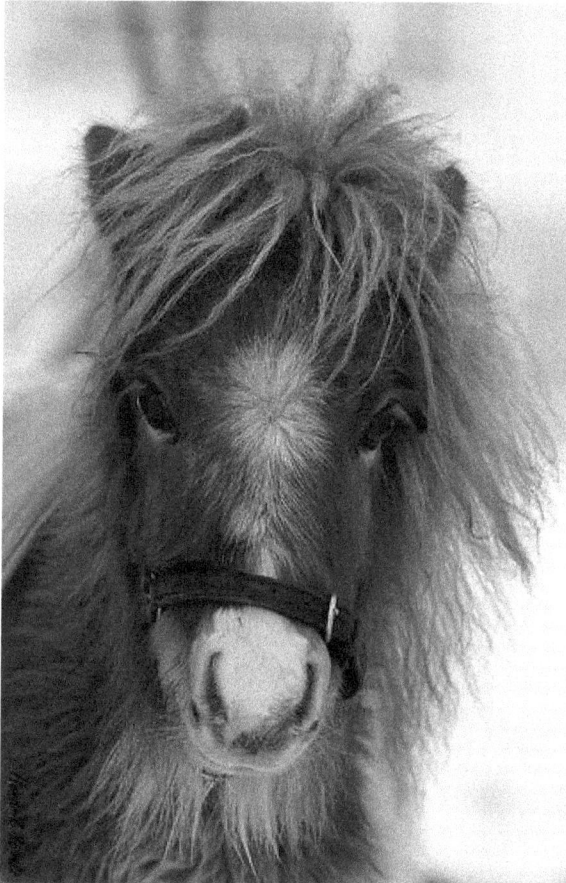

Vaccination is recommended against the Venezuelan strain (VEE) – especially for horses in southern U.S. states, especially those bordering Mexico.

Vaccination and mosquito control are important in helping prevent this disease.

Equine Influenza

Equine Influenza (inn- flu- en- zah) – is also known as the flu.

Influenza is a common disease caused by an influenza virus. This virus is easily spread from horse to horse through direct contact or contact with contaminated objects- such as food and water buckets, boots, grooming equipment and tack- and the hands of humans.

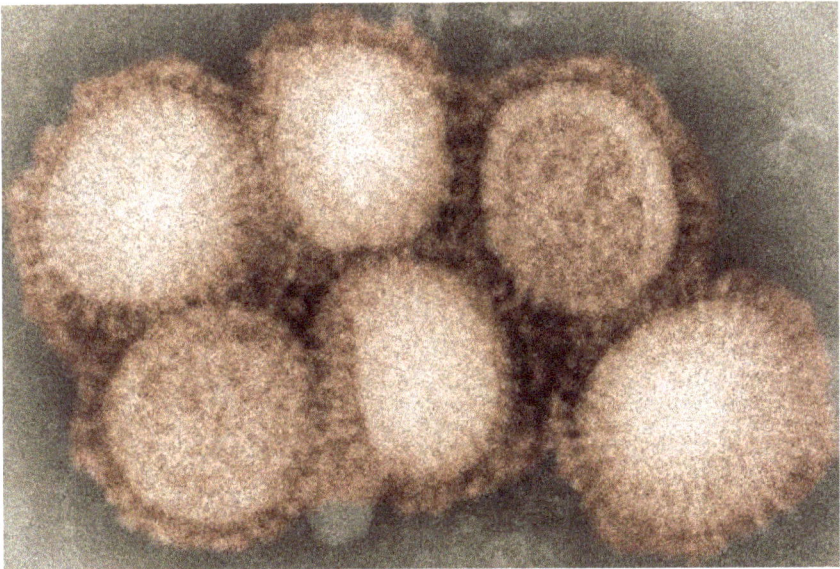

Equine influenza virus – visualized by electron microscopy

The reason influenza is a constant threat to horses is that the virus changes into new strains over time, and the protection the horse makes to the older form of the virus does not protect against the newer forms.

Signs of flu include:

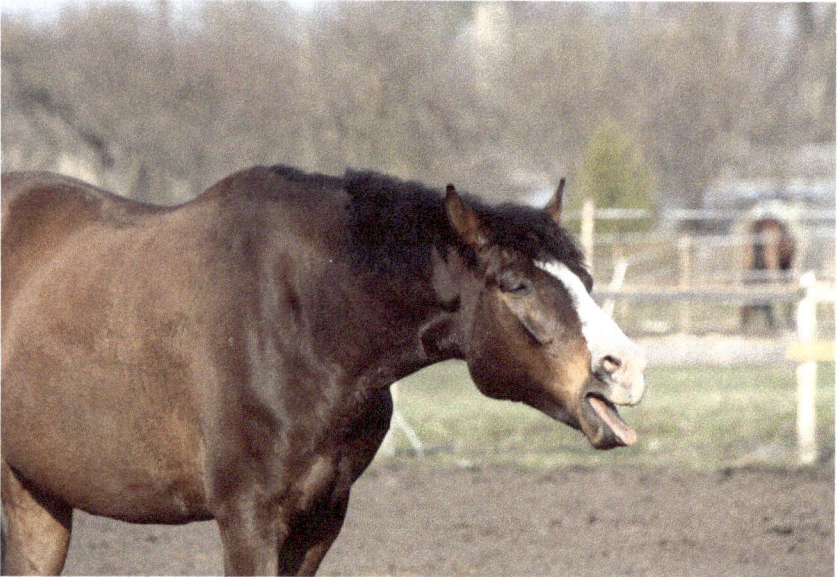

- fever
- coughing – that is harsh, dry and hacking that may last 2-3 weeks
- weakness
- depression
- watery or mucoid discharge from the nose that is yellow, tan, white or green, and
- loss of appetite

Infection with equine influenza is rarely fatal but can cause problems such as emphysema, pneumonia or bronchitis.

Flu has a short incubation (time from infection to signs of disease) time so it may appear suddenly, is costly to treat, and may leave a horse in a weakened condition. Do not fear, equine influenza cannot be passed to or from horses and humans.

Infected horses should be kept at complete rest to avoid complications from secondary bacterial infections such as pneumonia.

Seek advice from your veterinarian for treatment recommendations.

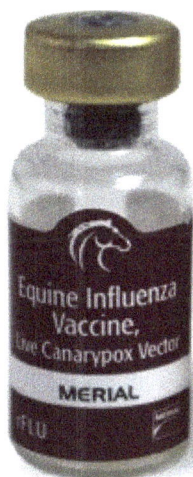

To avoid infection, it is best if newly arriving horses or horses that travel are separated from the other horses for at least 14 days.

All horses should receive a vaccine containing the most current influenza strains available before exposure. Sometimes more frequent vaccination is recommended for horses at high risk- such as show horses or race horses.

Streptcoccus Equi - (Strangles)

"Strangles" is a contagious disease seen most often in young horses and is caused by the bacteria *streptococcus equi* (strep- tow- cock-us ee-kweye). The name 'strangles' comes from the commonly seen abscessation (infection) of the tissue of the throat and neck areas.

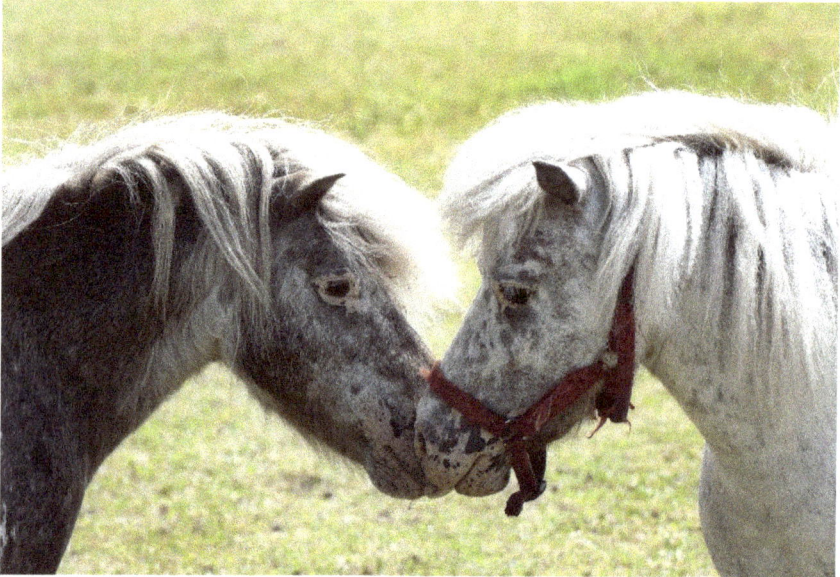

Strangles is transmitted by:

- direct contact with nasal secretions or pus from a draining sore from an infected horse
- contact with a sub- clinical shedder
- indirectly by contact with water troughs, hoses, feed buckets, pastures, stalls, trailers, tack, grooming equipment, cloths or sponges used for wiping horses' noses, caregiver's hands and clothing
- or insects such as flies contaminated with nasal discharge of an infected horse

Signs of strangles include:

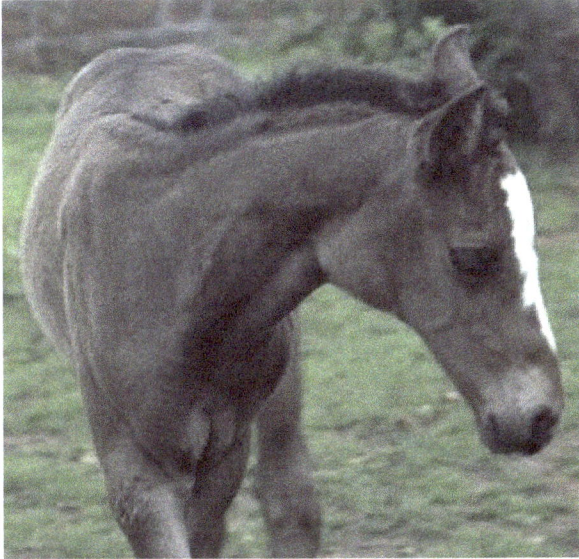

- fever (103°–106°F)
- nasal discharge that may be white, tan, yellow, or green
- depression
- difficulty swallowing
- respiratory noise that sounds harsh or rattle-like
- extension of the head and neck to make breathing easier
- swollen lymph nodes in the neck/throat area that may drain creamy white or yellow discharge

In addition to breathing difficulties and the signs above, in some outbreaks and, in a small percentage of horses, the abscesses spread to areas inside the horse (a condition known as 'bastard' strangles) which is nearly always fatal because the infection is not accessible and treatable when in the abdomen or chest of the horse.

As with other diseases, contact your veterinarian if you think your horse is showing signs of strangles. Treatment is essential.

Since strangles is easily spread to other horses, affected horses should be separated, and cared for by separate caretakers wearing protective clothing.

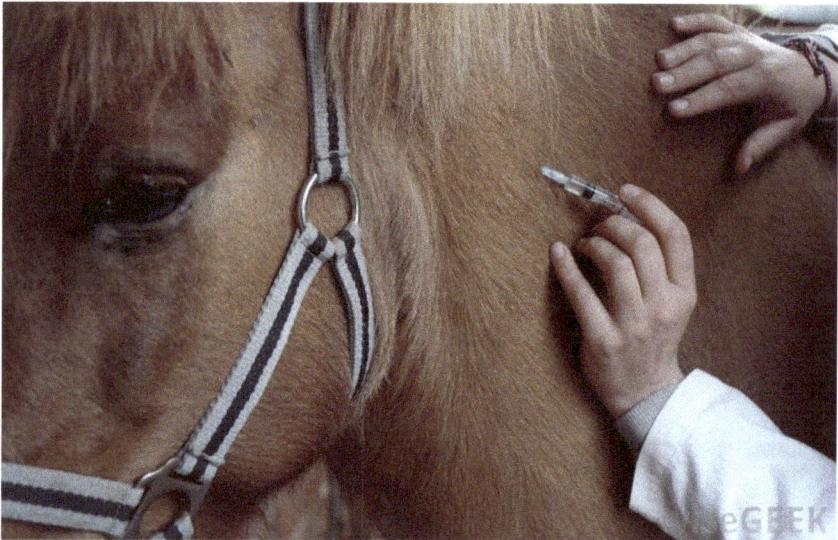

Vaccination is and effective way to prevent strangles. Contact your veterinarian for guidance.

Rhinopneumonitis/Equine Herpesvirus (EHV)

Rhinopneumonitis (Rye-no-new-mon-eye-tis) - AKA Equine Herpesvirus, 'rhino', and viral abortion virus - is a highly contagious respiratory disease caused by a virus that is spread through:

- aerosolized secretions (secretions in small particles in the air)
- contact with infected horses
- and contaminated feed and water utensils

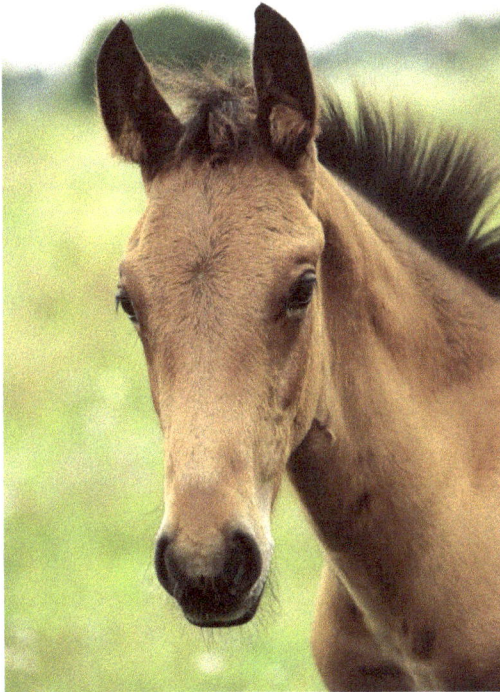

The 2 clinically important types of equine herpesvirus are EHV-1 and EHV-2

EHV-1 signs include: :

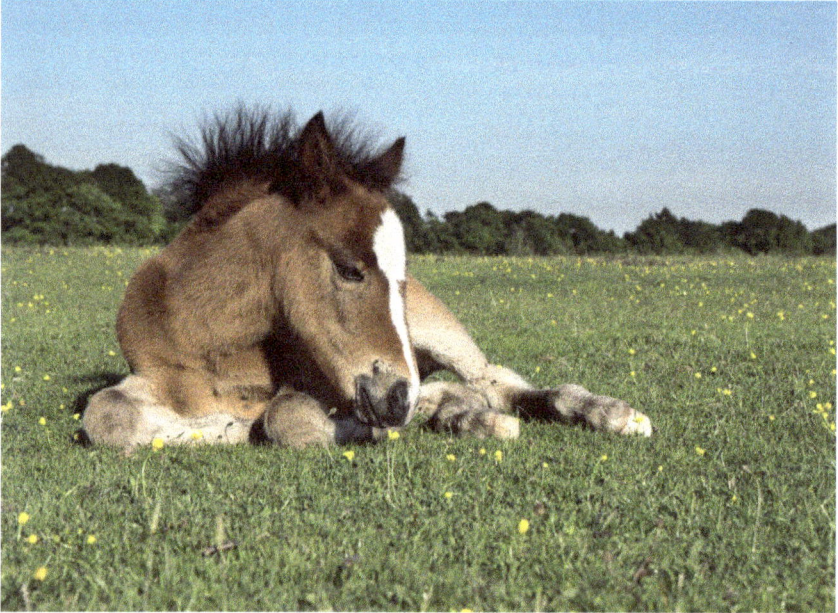

Respiratory disease - including -
- fever
- cough
- nasal discharge

Reproductive difficulties – such as -
- abortion or stillbirth of foals

Neurological issues (equine herpesvirus myeloencephalopathy)-
- mainly back leg weakness
- difficulty walking- incoordination – which may be seen as a horse leaning up against a fence for balance- and sometimes paralysis)
- depression
- urine dribbling
- head tilting
- inability to get up from the ground
- loss of ability to move their tail
- horses can be lost and vaccine is not available or effective

EHV-4 -signs are usually limited to respiratory signs including:

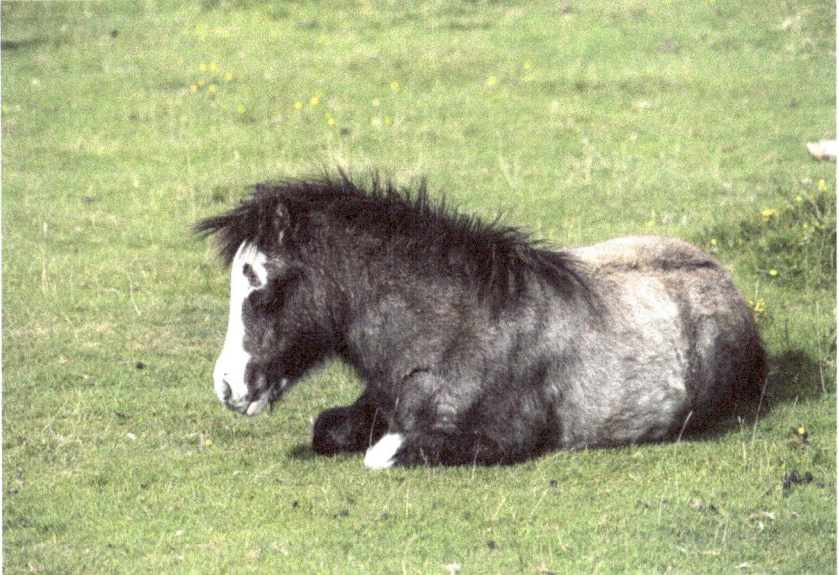

- nasal discharge
- cough
- noisy breathing and
- depression may be seen

Once a horse has been infected with EHV-1 or EHV-4, it will always be a carrier, and may shed the virus during times of stress.

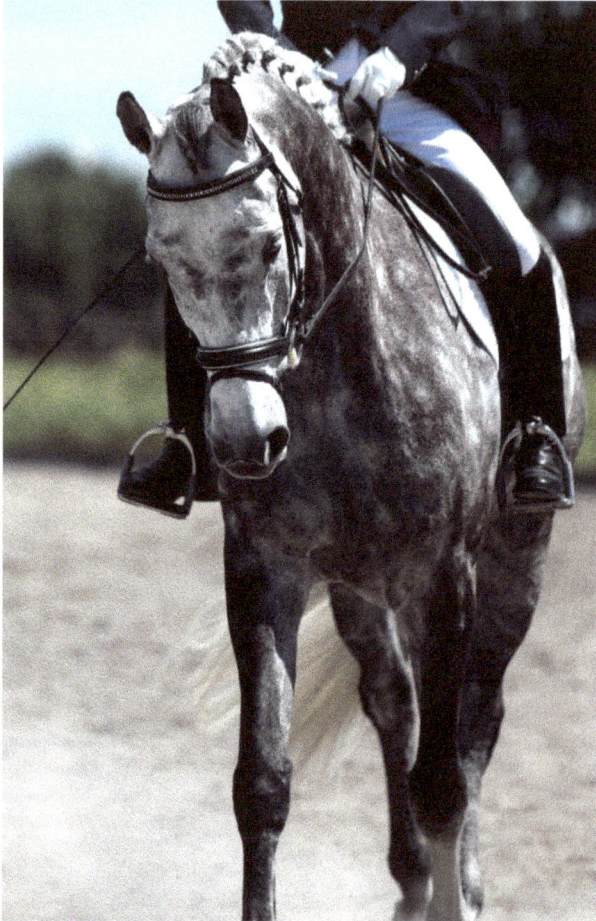

If you think your horse may have been exposed to the virus (while traveling or at a show) start isolation procedures immediately to prevent it from spreading through your whole herd.

In addition, check temperatures of all horses on your farm several times a day and, if fever is detected, check for EVH-1 and consult with your equine veterinarian for further guidance.

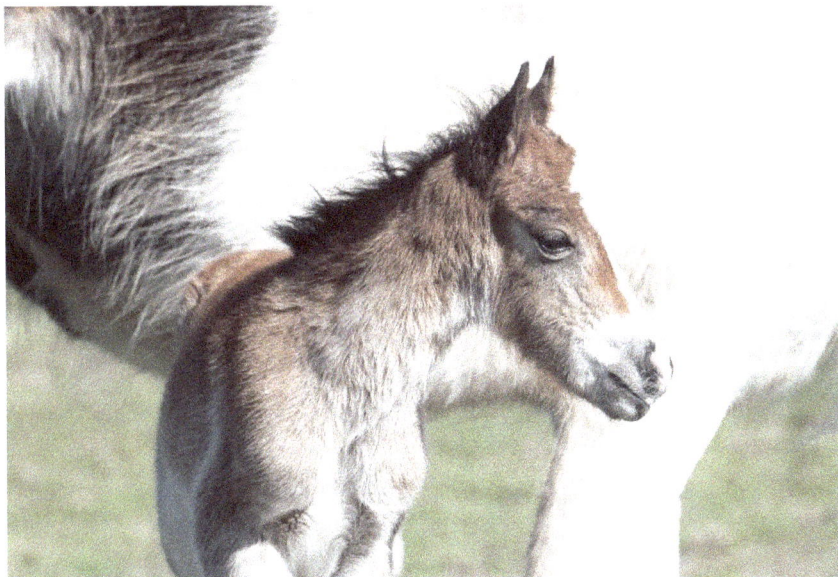

Prevention

Prevention on your farm is important and you can implement measures to minimize horses being exposed and becoming ill with rhinopneumonitis.

These practices include:

- quarantining any new animals on the farm
- as well as those that have traveled recently before introducing them to your herd
- washing instruments such as grooming supplies between use on each animal and limiting the use any equipment on multiple horses
- vaccinating every horse

Prevention: As stated, some repeated and additional ways to help prevent an EVH outbreak on your farm include:

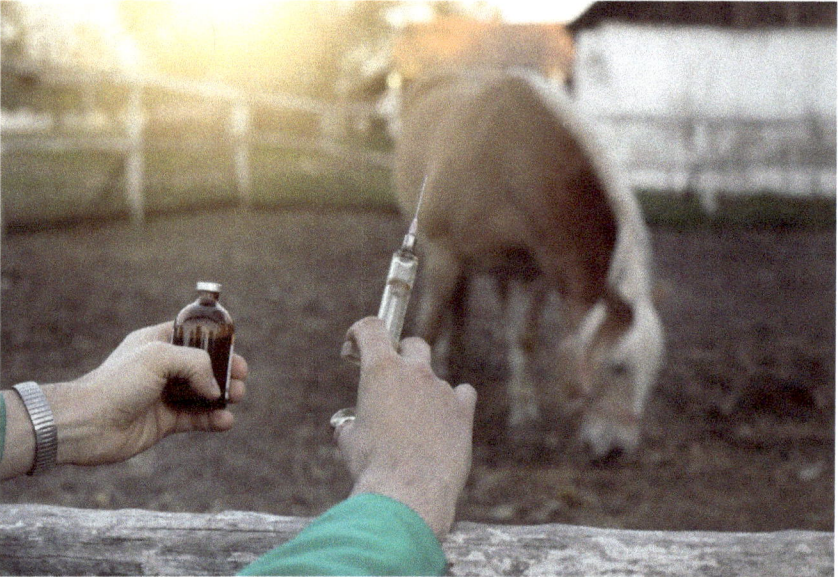

Every horse should be vaccinated for EHV-4 and EHV-1.

For abortion protection in the pregnant mare ask your veterinarian for vaccine recommendations.

Be aware! There is no licensed vaccine that has a claim for protection against the neurological strain of the herpes virus (equine herpesvirus myeloencephalopathy) noted previously.

Consult with your veterinarian for further guidance.

West Nile Virus

West Nile Virus – (WNV) causes disease in horses. The virus is transmitted to horses bitten by an infected mosquito.

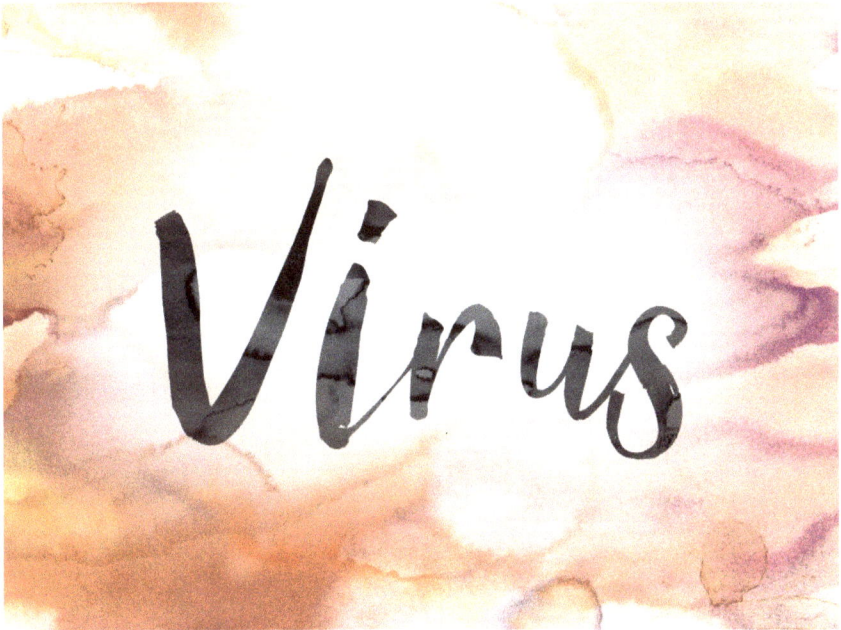

WNV circulates in nature between birds and mosquitoes. The virus is not transmitted from horse to horse or from horse to human, it can only be transmitted by a mosquito that has taken a blood meal from an infected bird. The horse or human affected cannot transmit the virus back to a mosquito that has bitten them.

Signs of West Nile Virus include:

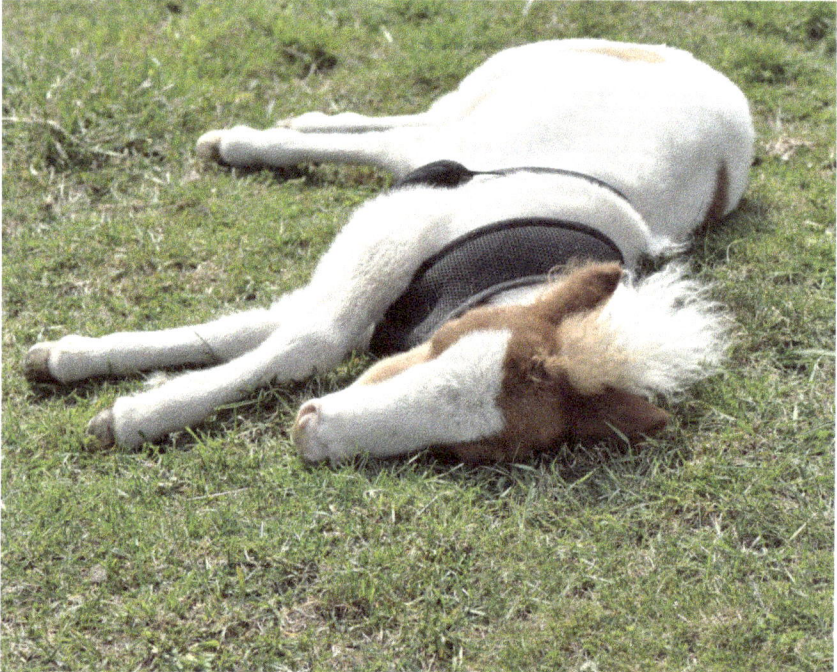

- no signs and the horse recovers on their own
- others may show signs that vary in range and severity, the most frequently observed signs include:
- depression or
- exaggerated response to stimuli such as noise or light in the environment
- fever

and…

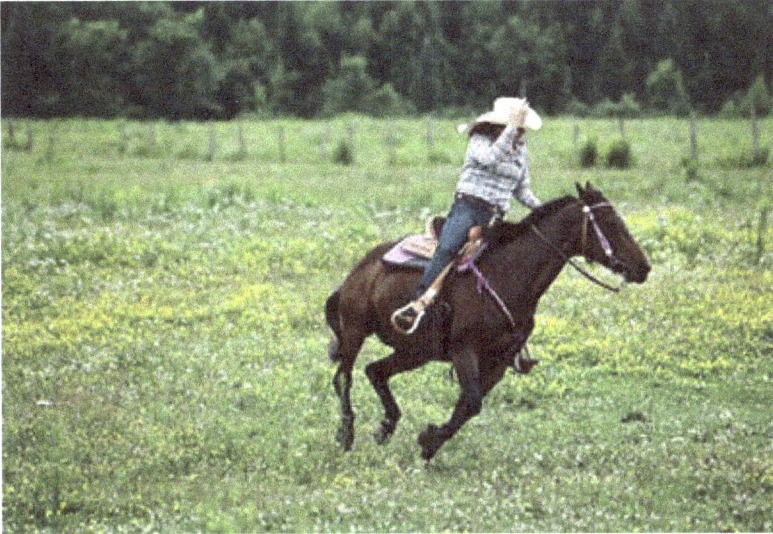

- weakness
- impaired vision
- infection that affects the brain and spinal cord (encephalomyelitis) causes lack of coordination – stumbling, falling, toe dragging, or leaning to one side or the other
- head pressing
- aimless wandering
- disorientation
- hyperexcitability
- drooping of the lower lip
- muscle twitching
- grinding teeth
- seizures
- inability to swallow
- excessive sweating
- and coma with loss of the horse

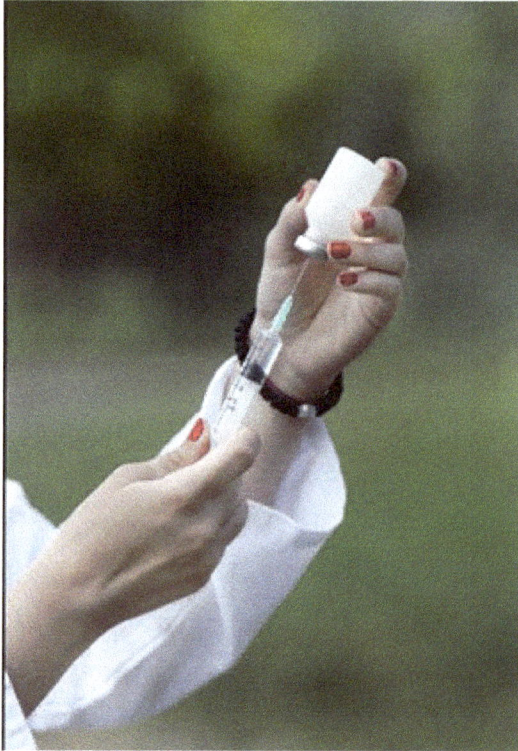

Prevention- it is recommended to vaccinate all horses at risk.

Quarantining horses is not necessary because a horse cannot transmit this disease directly to another horse.

.

Tetanus (Lockjaw)

Tetanus (lockjaw)- is a devastating disease caused by the bacteria *Clostridium tetani* which can be found in soil and manure.

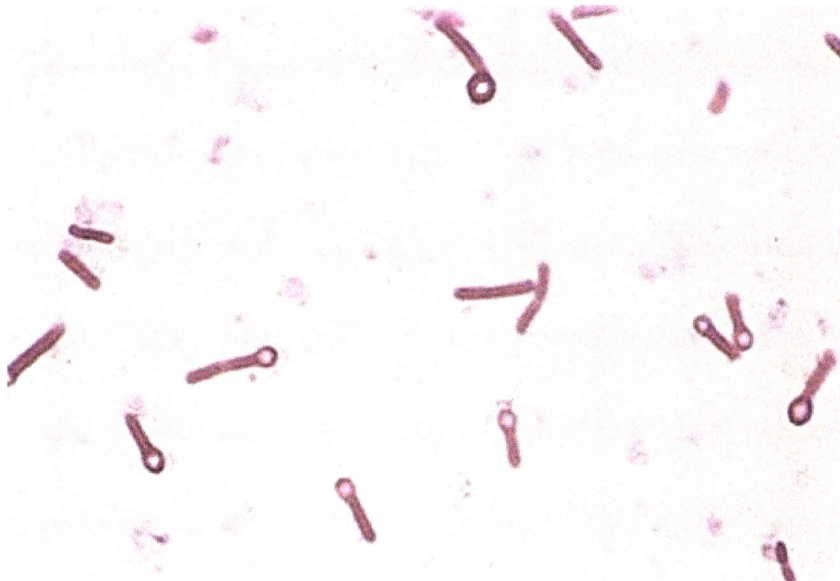

Clostridium tetani bacteria

These bacteria are found in every environment, and can survive for extended periods of time. Therefore, every horse should be vaccinated for tetanus because all are at risk if they experience a wound that may go undetected. Wound contamination is generally what leads to infection.

Clostridium tetani bacteria may enter wounds from –

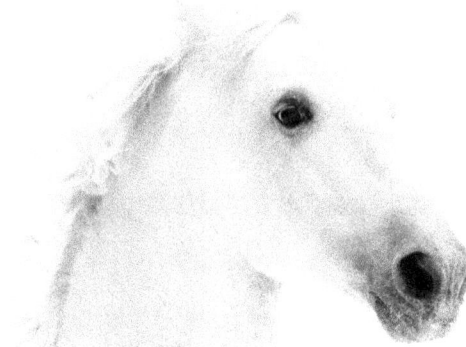

- barbed wire
- dropped nails
- surgical procedures such as castration
- cuts and deep puncture wounds
- or where a wound has healed over (such as the navel stump of a newborn foal) is an area where tetanus can thrive

Signs of tetanus include:

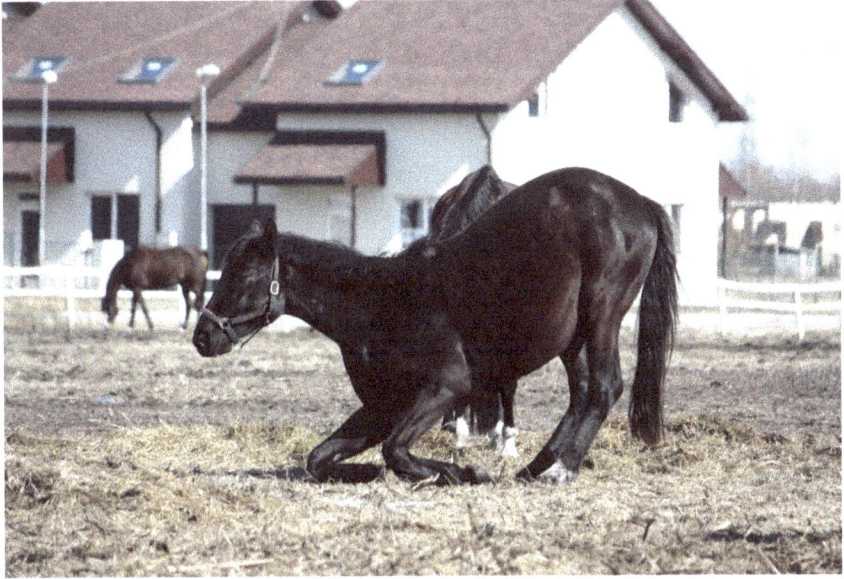

- stiff muscles
- or spasms of the muscles
- prolapsing of their third eyelid
- difficulty moving
- fever
- violent reactions to sudden movement or noise
- inability to eat
- holding the tail straight out
- standing in a 'sawhorse' manner
- sweating
- progressing to an anxious expression due to facial spasms and pain
- in advanced infection, the horse will collapse, seizure, and will be lost due to the inability to breath

Tetanus is often fatal.

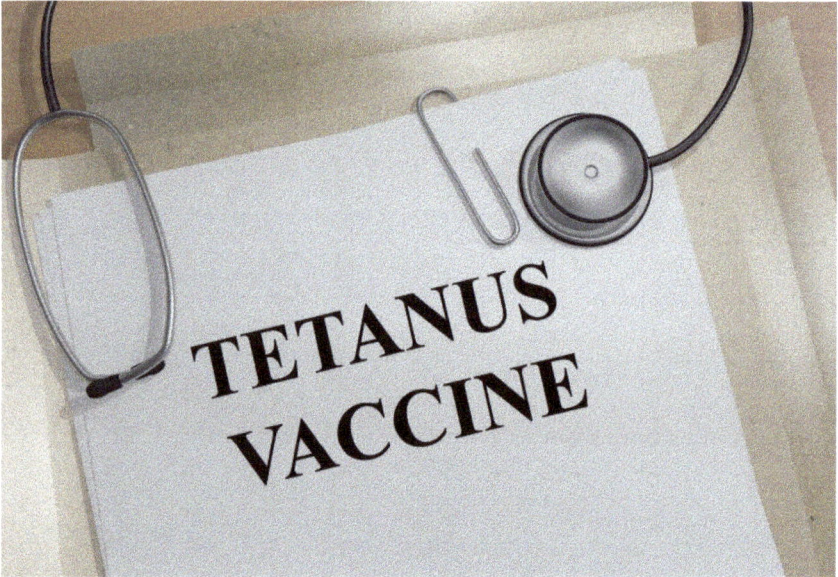

Tetanus vaccine is available and recommended in ALL horses to protect against this devastating disease.

Equine Rabies

Rabies is an incurable and fatal viral disease in warm blooded animals that is contracted from the bite of an infected animal.

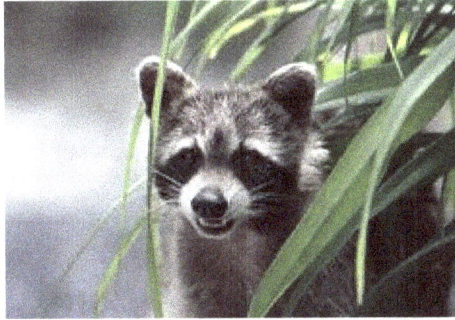

It is spread primarily by the bite of raccoons, bats, skunks, foxes and coyotes. Rabies may be seen anywhere in the US

Signs of rabies in horses include:

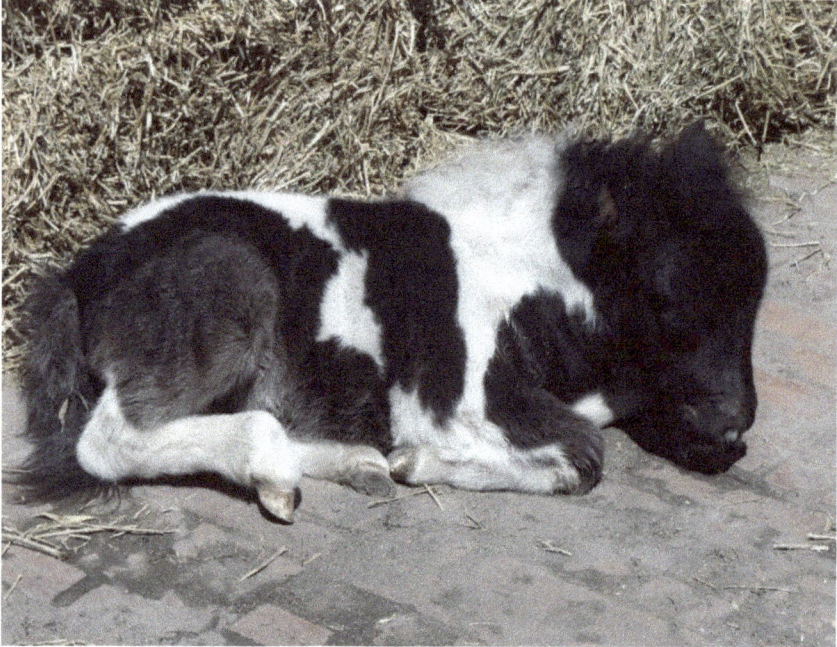

- neurological signs- seen as behavior changes, the inability to swallow, a head tilt, facial paralysis – drooping lips, and seizures are all possible
- uncoordinated gait- stumbling, wobbly gait
- weakness or paralysis that is worse in the rear legs
- excessive salivation
- fever
- occasionally bladder distention or dribbling urine
- occasionally horses may appear to have colic
- or a vague limping gait
- or tail weakness

If rabies is suspected, call a veterinarian immediately.

There are 2 forms of rabies

FURIOUS – this is a less common form and signs include:

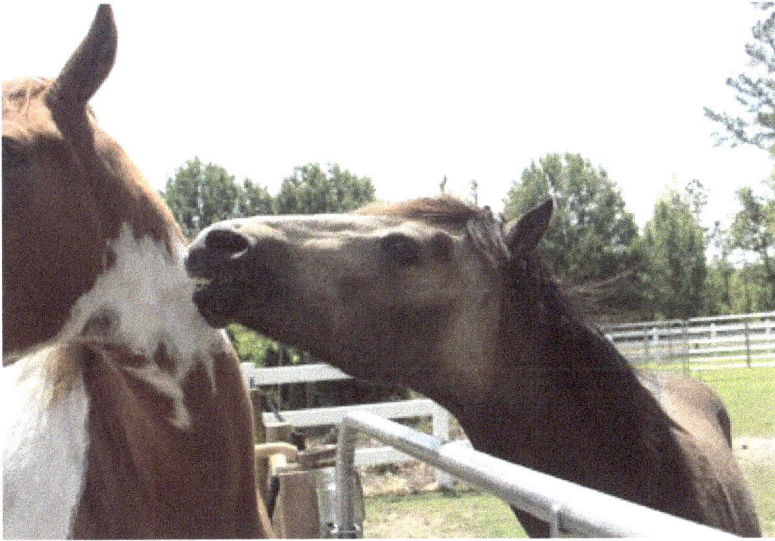

- a horse may become excitable
- fearful
- or aggressive – biting other animals or humans
- or may become increasingly sensitive to touch and light and other stimuli in the environment

DUMB or STUPOROUS – the more common form-signs include:

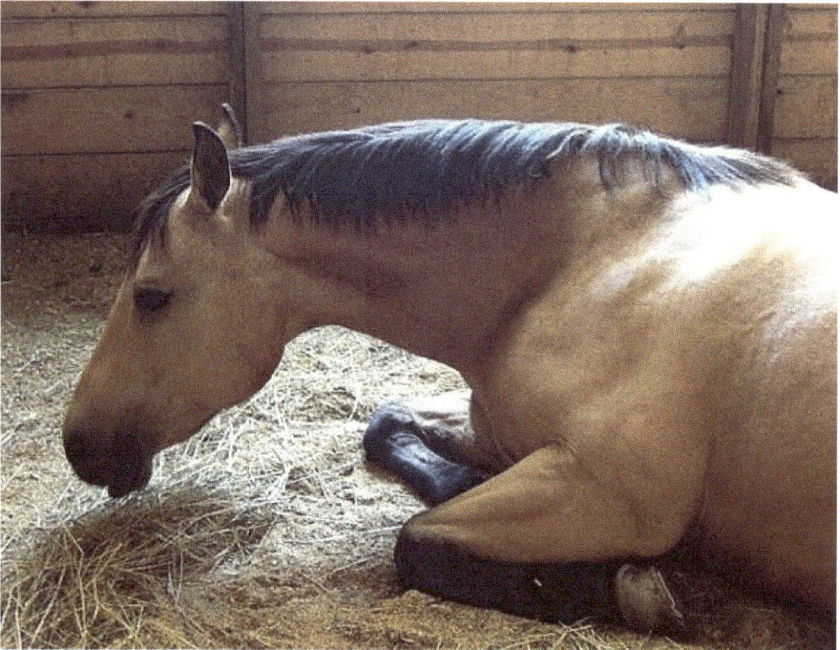

- depression
- loss of appetite
- pressing their head against the walls of the stall
- circling
- flaccid tongue, tail, and rectal area are possible

Rabies can be confused with many other horse diseases.

The danger in rabies is that humans are at risk as well. Rabies can be transmitted by exposure to the saliva of an infected horse as well as being bitten by an infected horse so, when rabies is suspected, you should avoid placing your hands in the mouth of a suspect horse. Call a veterinarian immediately.

There is no treatment for rabies.

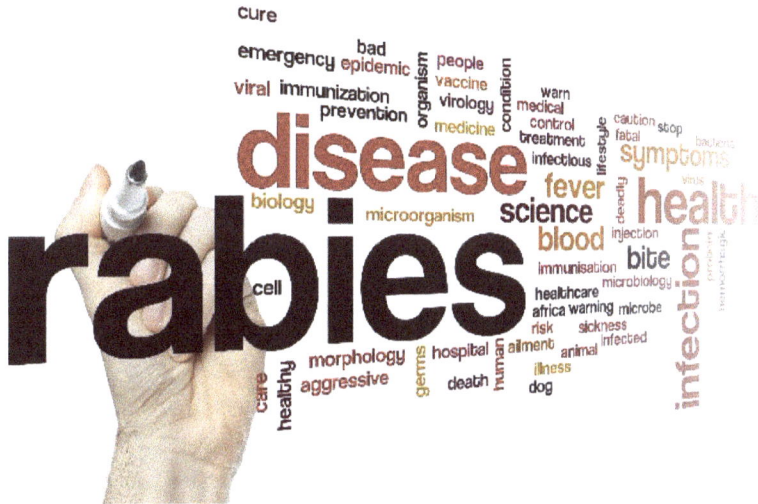

Since there is no treatment for rabies, health departments and governments around the country recommend and may require vaccinating all eligible animals for rabies. As noted, rabies is a disease that may affect humans.

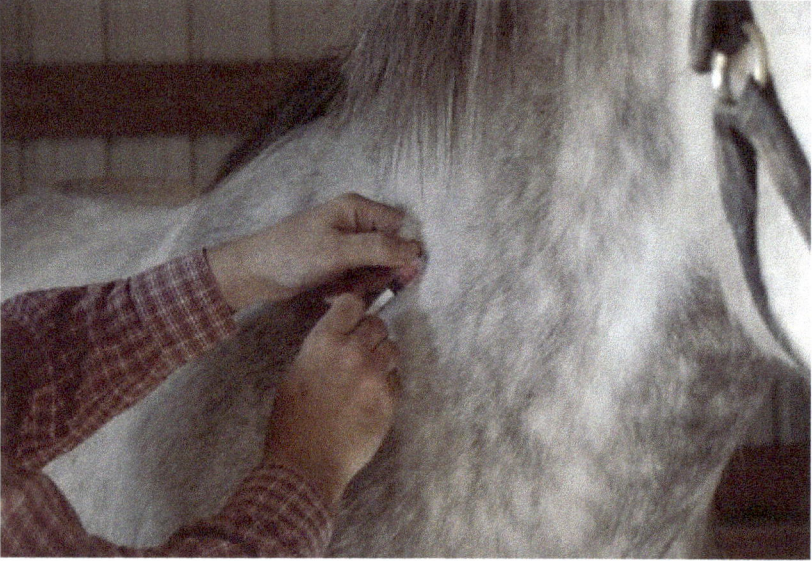

Rabies vaccine is available and recommended for all horses.

Potomac Horse Fever (PHF)

Potomac Horse Fever- is a bacterial infection of the blood and tissues of horses. It is caused by *Neorickettsia risticii*, which is found in flatworms that develop in aquatic snails.

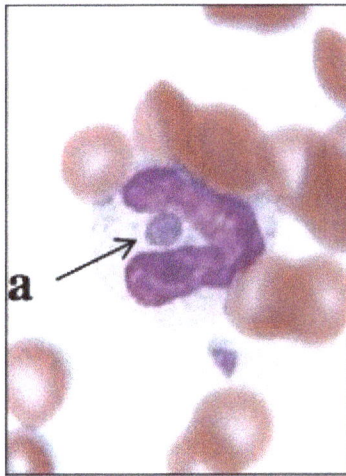

Named after the region where the disease was first diagnosed in 1979, this disease. is much more common in spring, summer and early fall and is only found in certain areas of the country – the northern US and Canada- and is associated with pastures bordering water sources such as creeks or rivers

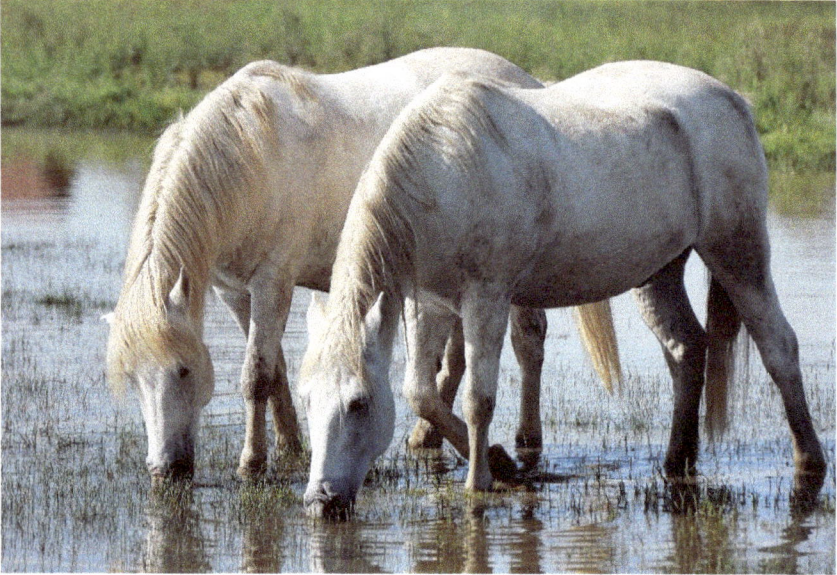

When the water warms, infected immature flatworms are released from snails into the water. These immature flatworms may be ingested by horses drinking the water, but more commonly they are picked up by water insects. Infected insects (such as mayflies) hatch and carry the organism to horses to ingest as they graze.

.

Signs of Potomac Horse Fever include:

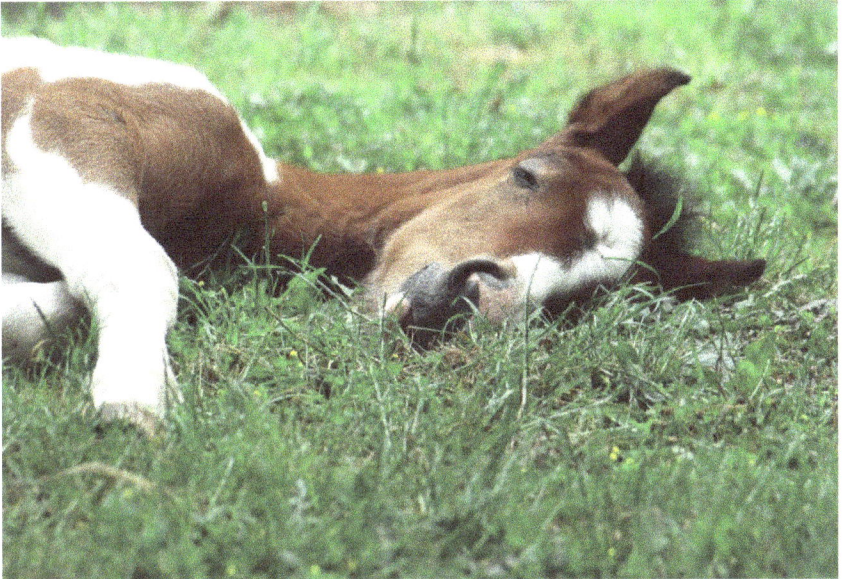

- mild symptoms to
- fever
- loss of appetite
- depression
- decrease in the intestinal sounds (stomach rumbling)
- mild colic (abdominal pain)
- lameness
- diarrhea that is usually profuse and watery that can lead to
- laminitis (a serious condition where the hoof wall begins to separate from the bones of the foot (see cpt 8) and
- dehydration,
- shock
- and occasionally death
- potomac horse fever also causes abortion of foals in pregnant mares

If you think your horse is showing signs of Potomac horse fever you should contact your veterinarian immediately.

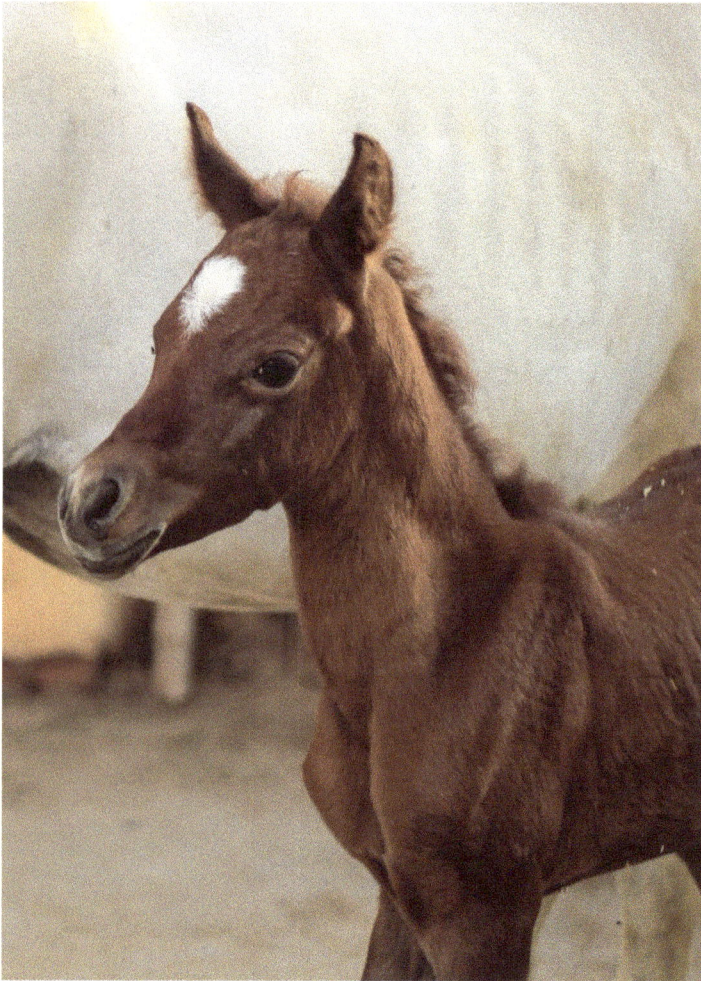

PHF is easily diagnosed by laboratory identification of the organism in a blood or manure sample. If caught early, it can be treated successfully,

Vaccination is strongly recommended for horses in areas where Potomac horse fever has been diagnosed and for horses traveling to such areas- such as Maryland, Eastern Virginia or other areas. Show horses may encounter horses from these areas. Vaccination may not completely prevent illness, but may reduce its severity if the horse is exposed to the organism.

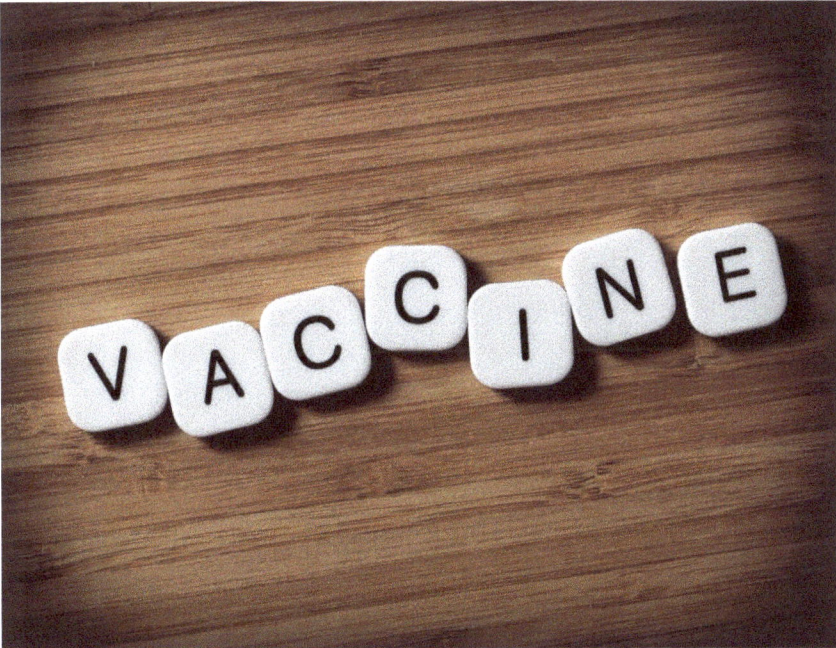

Consult with your veterinarian to decide the best course of action.

Equine Protozoal Myeloencephalitis (EPM)

Equine Protozoal Myeloencephalitis – (EPM) (pro- toe- zoe- all my-ell- oh-en – cef- ah- lie- tis)- is an infection of the nervous system (the brain and spinal cord) of horses.

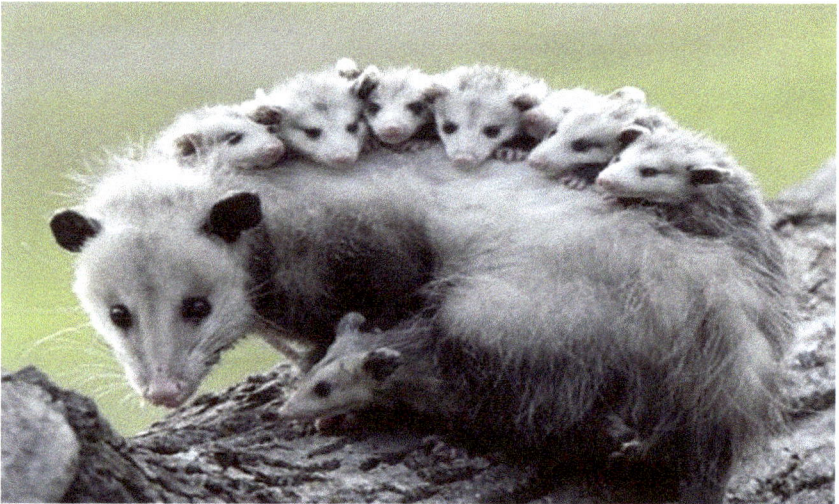

The opossum has been implicated as the definitive host of the EPM organism.

Signs of EPM include:

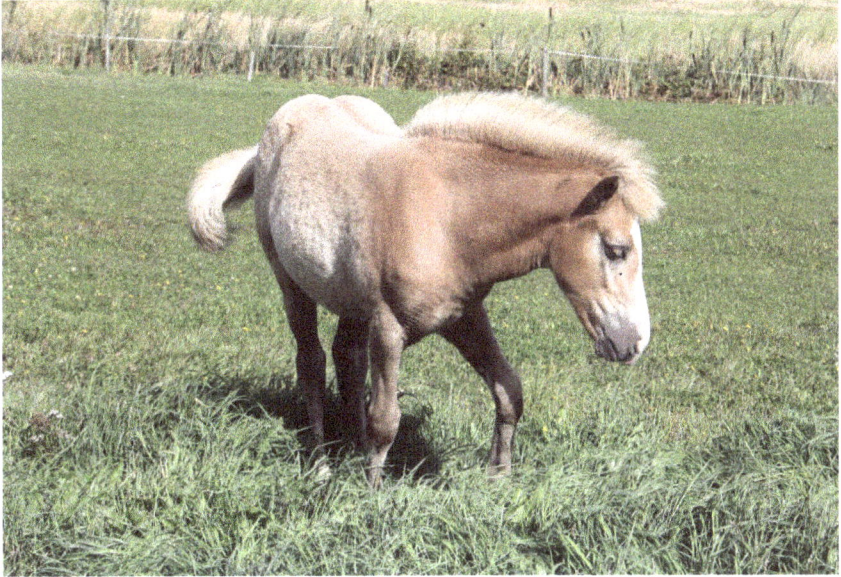

- neurologic signs such as
- incoordination (ataxia)
- weakness
- spasms of the muscles
- inability to walk
- unable to rise when lying down

TESTING - Any horse suspected of having EPM should have his/her cerebrospinal fluid (CSF- the fluid around the brain and spinal cord) tested for the presence of antibodies to this parasite.

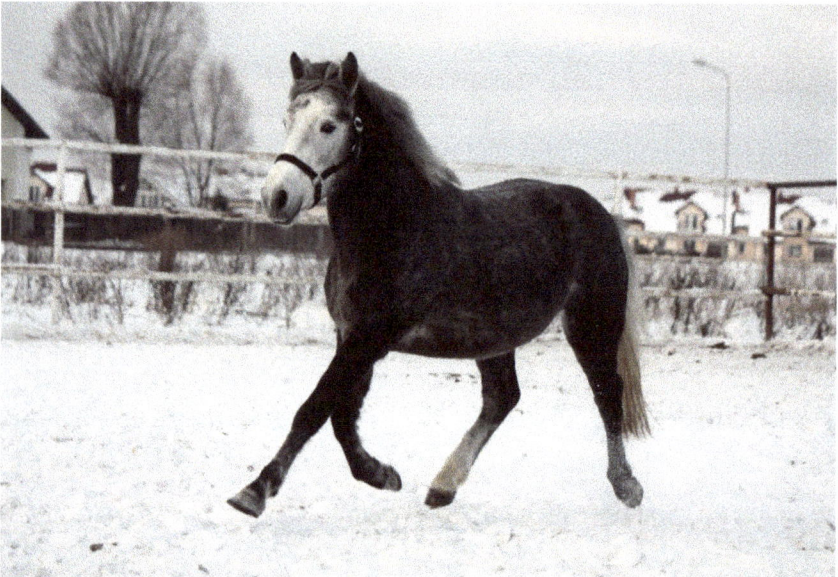

Currently, there is no effective vaccine for EPM.

Equine Infectious Anemia Virus (EIA)

Equine Infectious Anemia Virus (EIA)- is a potentially fatal viral disease that there is no cure or effective treatment for.

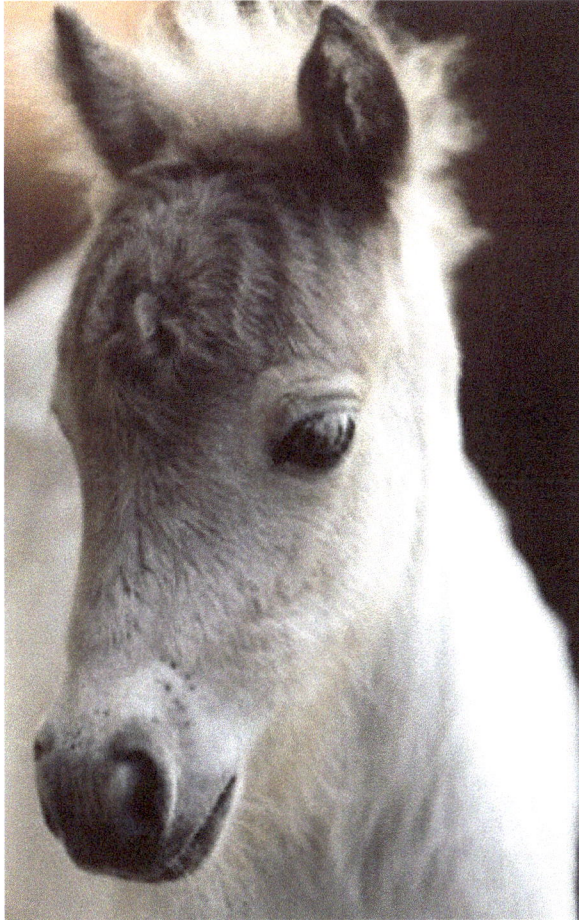

EIA virus is transmitted by blood exposure or by passage across the placenta in the pregnant mare directly to the foal. Blood transmission can occur via blood-sucking insects such as horse flies, deer flies and mosquitoes.

Signs of EIA include:

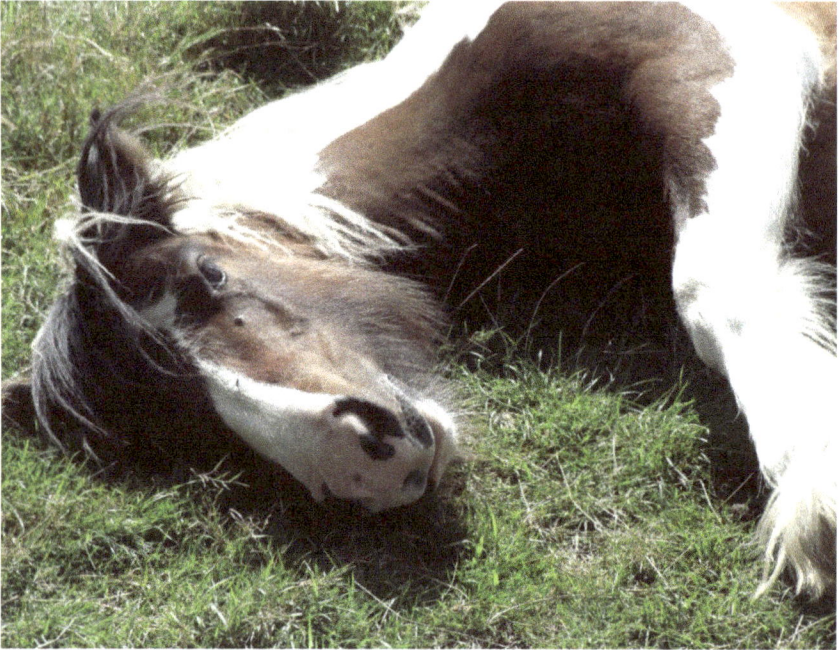

- no signs, but are still able to spread the disease for life – endangering the health of other horses
- fever
- depression
- decreased appetite
- decreased stamina/weakness
- rapid weight loss

Equine Infectious Anemia is a reportable disease to the proper health authorities.

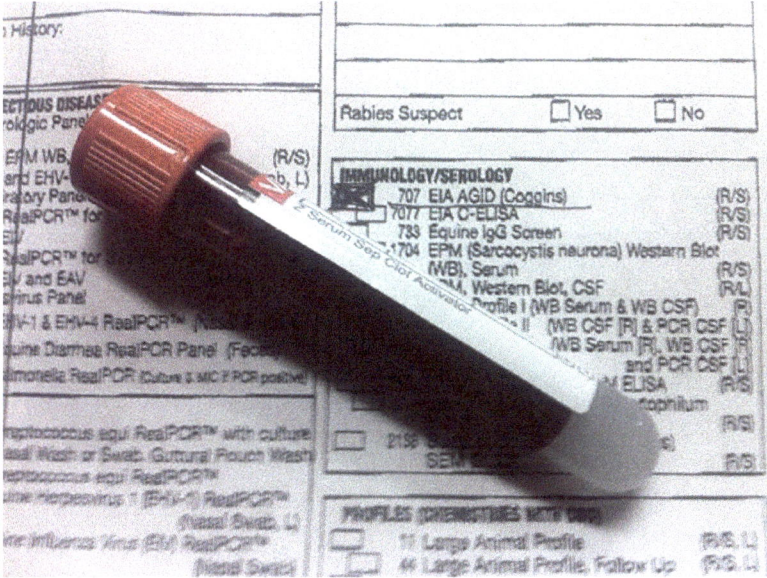

The Coggins test is the only way to accurately determine whether a horse is infected. All positive cases must be filed with the State veterinarians and the Federal Animal and Plant Health Inspection Service. Your veterinarian will help with this.

If your horse tests positive for EIA, your options are extremely limited for care or sale or movement of the horse.

Vaccine reactions

Yes, vaccines prevent disease or lessen the severity of disease. They lower the cost of care for pets.

Most of the time one cannot even tell a pet has received a vaccine, however …......

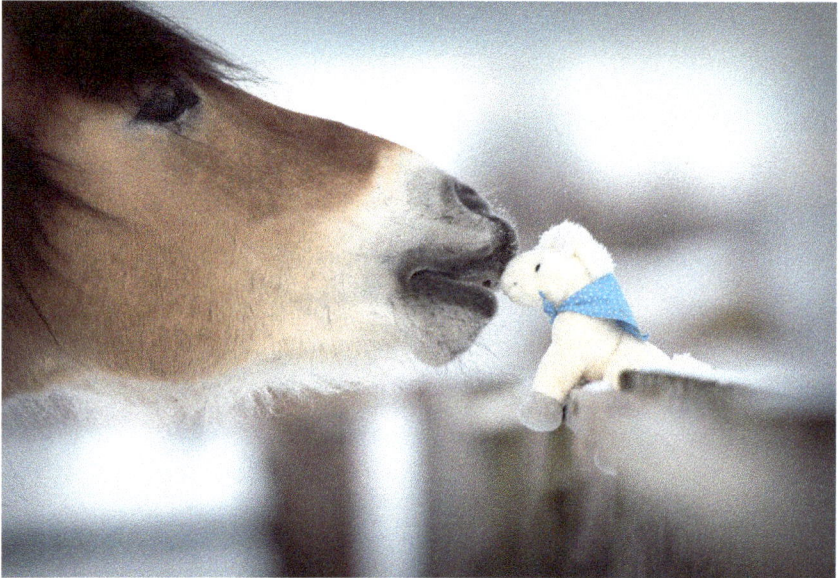

.....adverse reactions to vaccines can occur. These reactions are uncommon, however, can be alarming and even devastating.

Reactions range from mild soreness at the injection site to not exercising or eating/drinking as well for 1-2 days after being vaccinated.

More severe reactions include:

1. swelling and soreness at the injection site
2. fever
3. swelling to a limb
4. loss of appetite

Severity of signs may progress to anaphylaxis, which includes:

1. laminitis
2. systemic shock
3. difficulty breathing
4. staggering
5. seizures
6. inability to walk
7. coma
8. loss of pet

All adverse signs/symptoms noted by owners should be taken seriously and reported to their veterinarian, and if your veterinarian is not available, you should have your pet seen at an emergency clinic for horses.

Reactions can be frightening to owners and may discourage vaccinating. If a pet has experienced an adverse reaction to a vaccine, or an owner would like to prevent reactions in high-risk pets, veterinarians may recommend pre-treating pets prior to vaccinating to reduce or eliminate the risk of an adverse reaction from occurring.

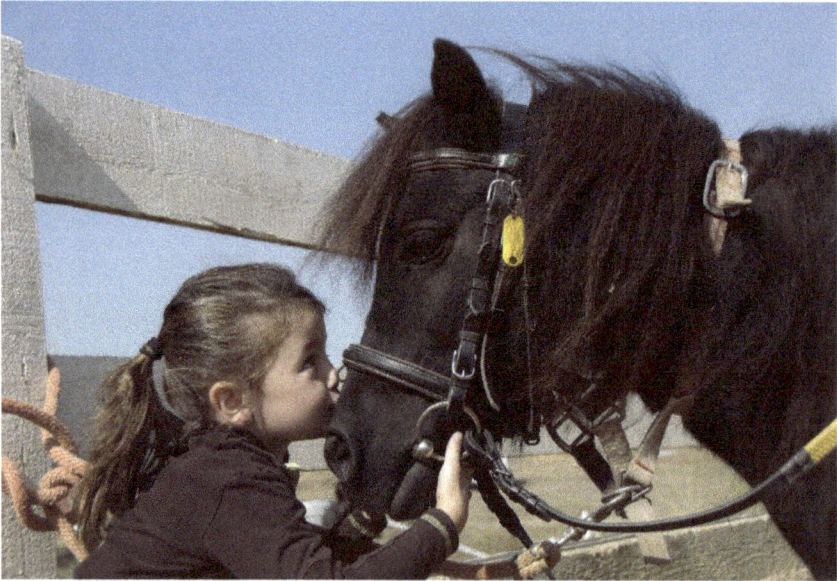

Horses are at extreme risk if not vaccinated. The profound consequences that may occur need to be discussed with your veterinarian. If you are one of the unfortunate owners with a horse that has reacted to a vaccine or vaccines, ask your veterinarian for recommendations. Some elect to:

- change the brand of vaccine
- change the site of vaccination
- give only 1 vaccine at a time
- exercise after vaccinating
- only vaccinate for necessary diseases – rabies and tetanus are strongly recommended for all horses
- if a horse is not fully vaccinated, keeping them away from other horses is recommended as well as fly and mosquito control is imperative

Chapter 3

Tick-Borne Diseases

Tick-Borne Diseases on the Rise: How to Protect Your Horse

Ticks can be difficult to detect because they range from a tiny size to a visible size. Ticks are opportunistic - many hide in dark places and wooded areas. They can climb tall grass to attach to horses and cause disease.

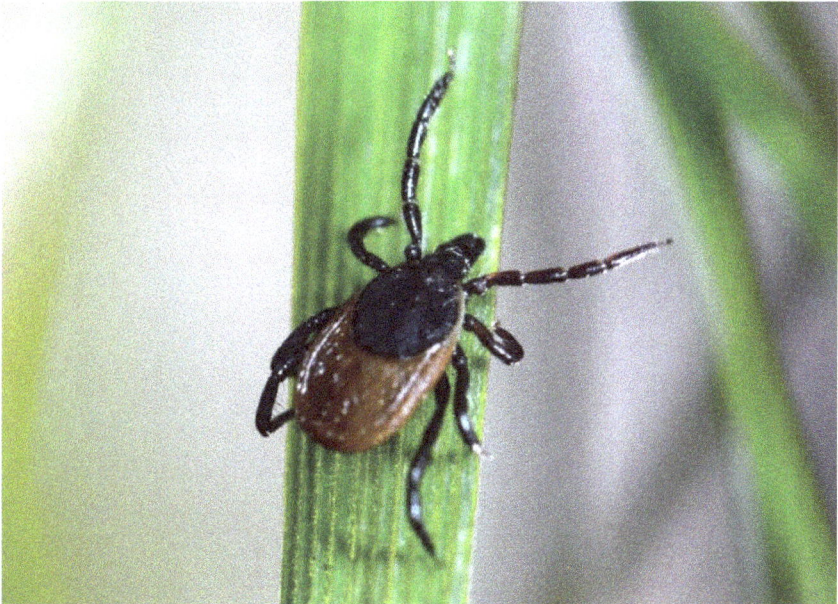

Although ticks are small, they are capable of transmitting bacteria, viruses, and blood parasites - some of which can be life-threatening, even deadly.

The good news is that there are easy ways to protect you and your horse from ticks and the diseases they transmit.

The three main tick-borne diseases that can affect horses are:

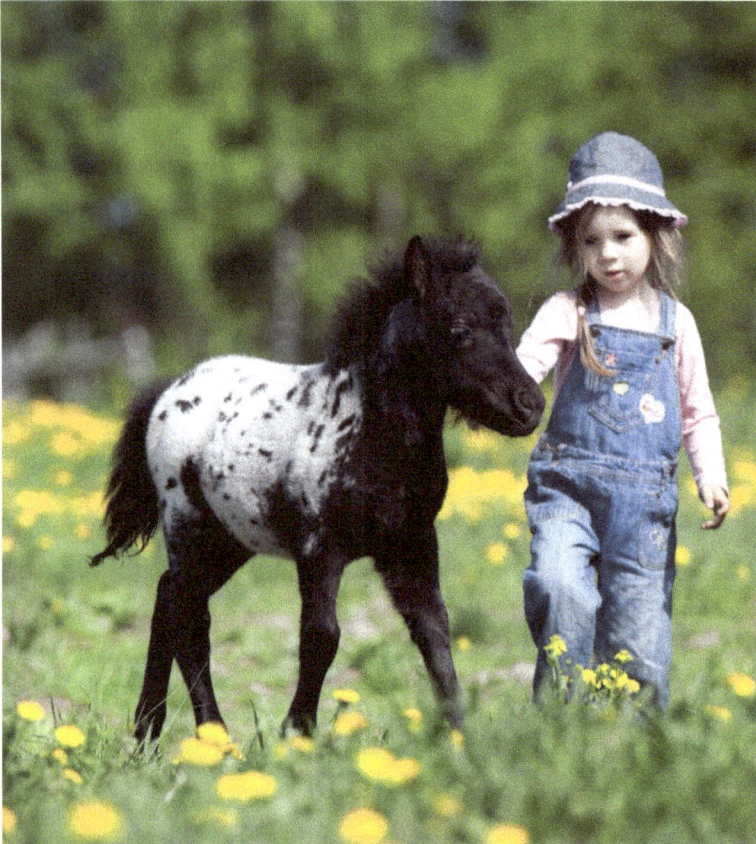

- Lyme disease
- Equine piroplasmosis
- Anaplasmosis

Diagnosis may be challenging because tick-borne diseases have many signs that are similar to other diseases which may be confusing as well as the tick may not remain on the horse.

Tick disease is not transferred from our horses to humans, but may occur in humans if exposed to the ticks the horse is exposed to.

Lyme disease

Lyme disease - is transmitted by ticks carrying the infective organism *Borrelia burgdorferi*.

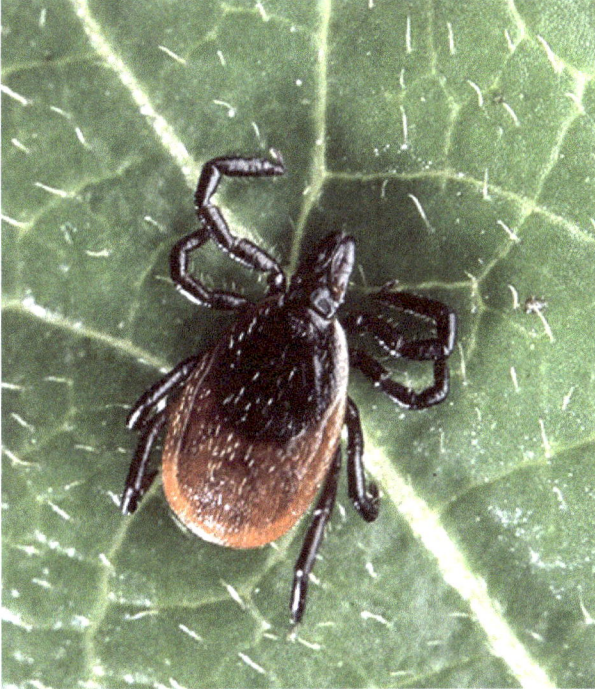

Lyme is transmitted by *Ixodes scapularis,* found in the north and eastern U.S. and *Ixodes pacificus*, found in the western U.S. They are known as "deer ticks" and "eastern or western black-legged ticks," respectively.

Lyme disease can affect humans as well as horses, dogs and cats.

Signs of Lyme disease include:

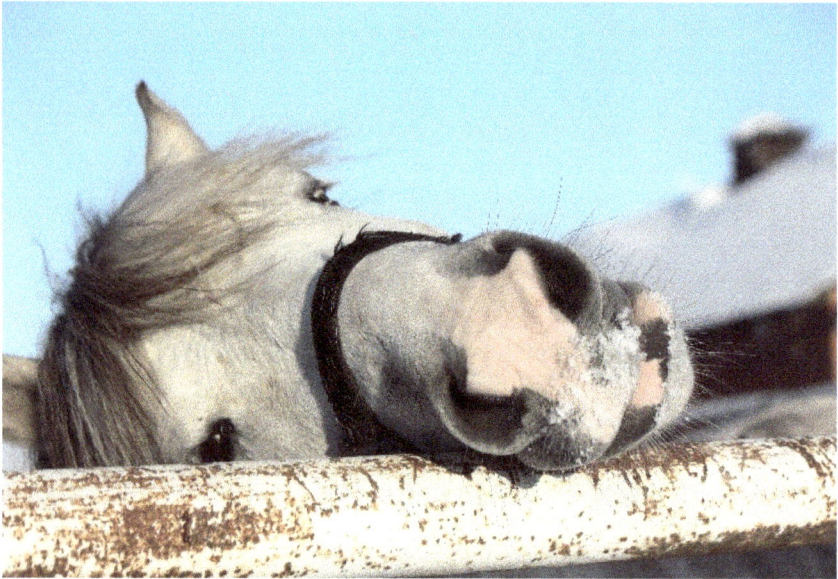

- no signs at all to
- muscle stiffness
- lameness (limping) in more than one leg
- muscle tenderness
- decrease muscle mass – muscle wasting
- weight loss
- depression or dullness
- behavioral changes such as disorientation or not responding to commands
- sensitive skin- making touching the horse painful
- severe signs include neuroborreliosis (disease of the nerves seen by inner eye irritation (uveitis)
- the joint swelling seen in dogs and humans is generally not seen in horses

Signs of Lyme disease may not appear for an extended time, or can appear shortly after the tick has fed on the horse.

Equine Piroplasmosis

Equine piroplasmosis (pie- row- plaz- moe- sis) is a blood cell infection with protozoal organisms- either *Babesia caballi* or *Theileria equi* (formerly called *Babesia equi*).

Babesia caballi

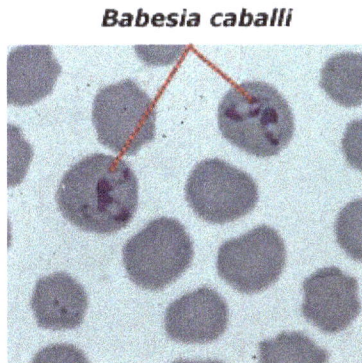

These blood parasites can be transmitted by several species of ticks.

It can take seven days to a month after the tick has fed on the horse for signs of equine piroplasmosis disease to appear.

Signs of piroplasmosis include:

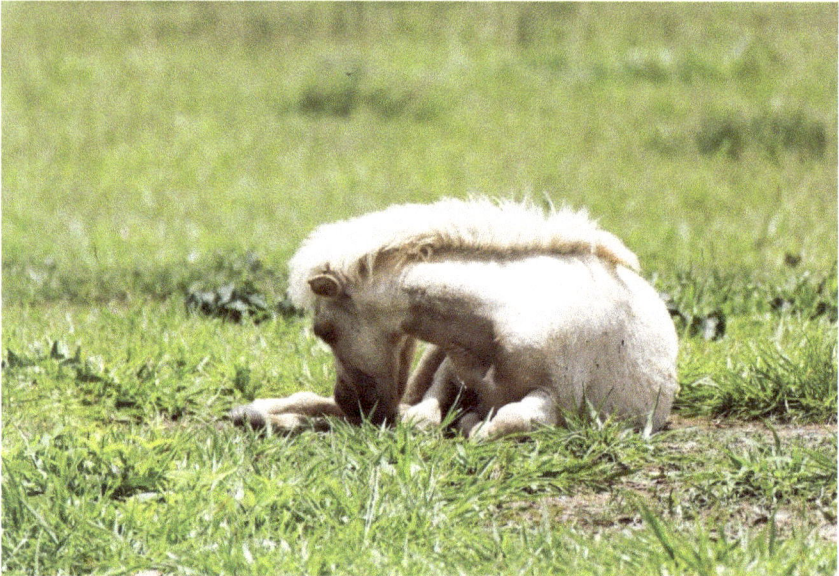

- few to no signs
- mild weakness
- depression
- fever (104F)
- fast but shallow breathing
- decreased appetite
- weight loss
- pale gums or
- jaundice (yellow coloring to the gums and eyes and skin)
- dark colored urine
- abortion of foals in pregnant mares
- swelling to the lower legs

Piroplasmosis is a reportable disease to State and Federal agencies.

Horses may be treated and have no signs of piroplasmosis, however, they will always be carriers of the disease.

Anaplasmosis

Equine granulocytic anaplasmosis (ana- plazz- moe- sis) -is a blood infection caused by *Anaplasma phagocytophilum.*

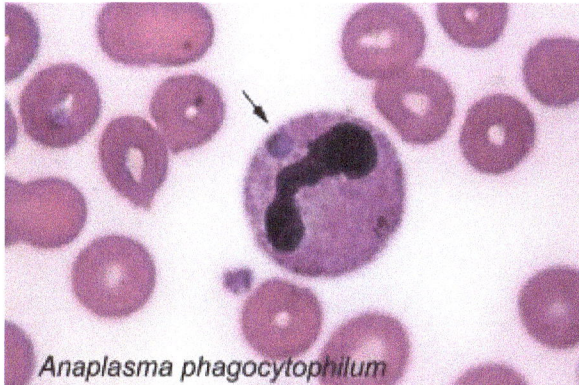

Anaplasma phagocytophilum

Anaplasmosis is transmitted by deer ticks like Lyme, but caused by different bacteria than that causing Lyme disease.

It tends to occur in young horses.

Signs usually don't appear until 8-14 days after exposure.

Signs of anaplasmosis include:

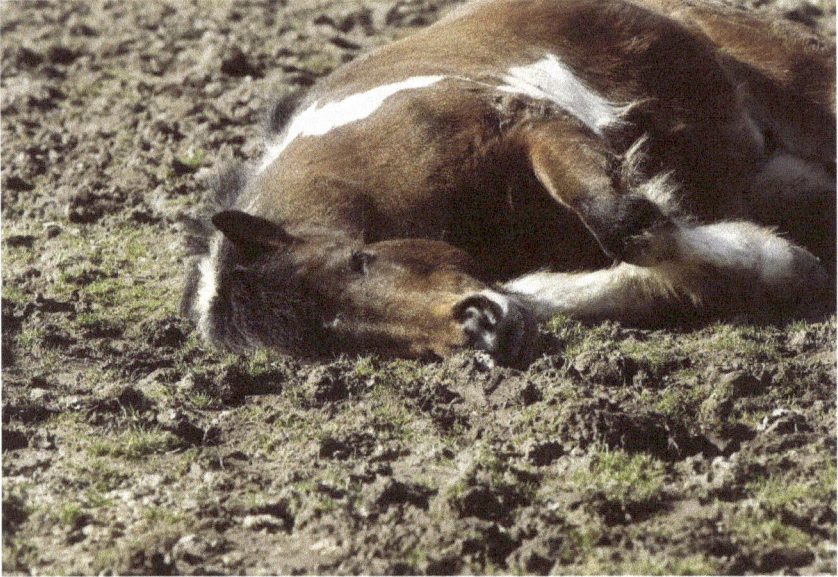

- fever (104F)
- depression
- decreased appetite
- swelling to the legs
- stumbling gait also sees as
- incoordination (ataxia)

Diagnosis for these diseases is made by blood testing.

Seek veterinary care for treatment recommendations.

Many veterinarians feel there are NO 'safe' ticks. New diseases are always being identified.

PREVENTION OF TICK DISEASE

Develop a Strategy

Currently there are no vaccines for tick-borne diseases in horses.

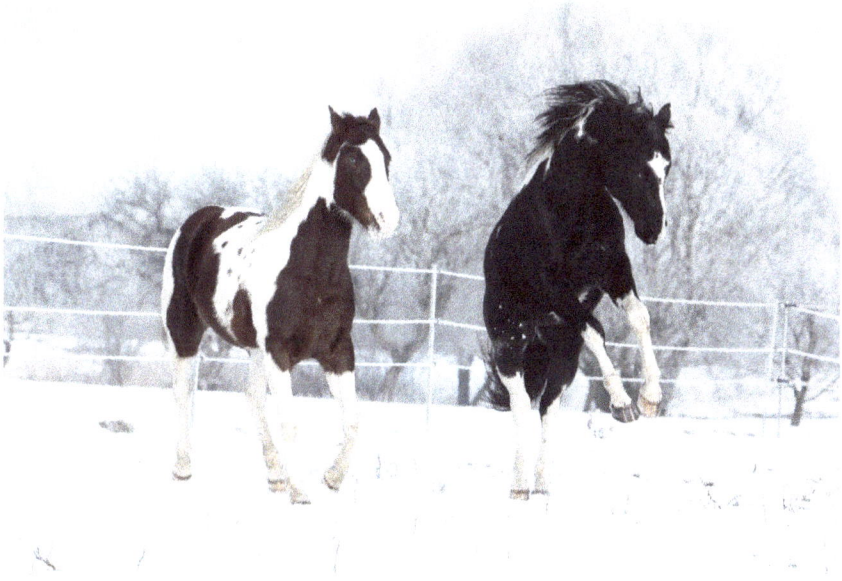

Important! Ticks are not just a warm weather concern. These hardy creatures can survive in winter, insulated in vegetation beneath snow. There is even one species, the "winter tick," that is only on horses during the cool seasons—even during sub-zero winter weather—and spends the summer away from animals.

PREVENTION OF TICK DISEASE INCLUDE:

- year-round prevention of ticks
- management – which includes avoiding tick exposures, treating the premises, and treating the horses specifically
- since ticks thrive in protective layers of vegetation and tall grasses, one of the best ways to avoid tick exposure is to limit or prevent access to wooded areas, including the boundaries to such wooded areas
- keep pastures mowed to prevent excessively tall grass, and clear brush from around fence lines- ticks usually avoid crossing hot, sunny areas with little vegetation
- some horse owners hire a pest control company to spray along the wooded areas to create a chemical barrier - it can also be a benefit to have a fresh set of eyes to help find problem areas on your property
- to protect the horses themselves, apply an approved product specifically for ticks made for use on horses- read the whole label, including the warning section, before applying and if you have a foal, make certain the product is approved for use on young animals- spot-on liquid products are most commonly used for pastured horses and these horses are ideal candidates for such a product when you can't groom them daily and check for ticks
- if you do find a tick on your horse- remove it with tweezers or a tick removal tool, grasping the tick by its mouthparts as close to the horse's skin as possible - don't twist or jerk; just pull it out with steady, even pressure and don't squeeze the tick's body

Seek recommendations for tick prevention from your veterinarian.

Chapter 4

Castrating Horses

Rarely do veterinarians remove ovaries in mares. On the rare occasion this surgery is performed, it is usually because one or both ovaries are enlarged or diseased.

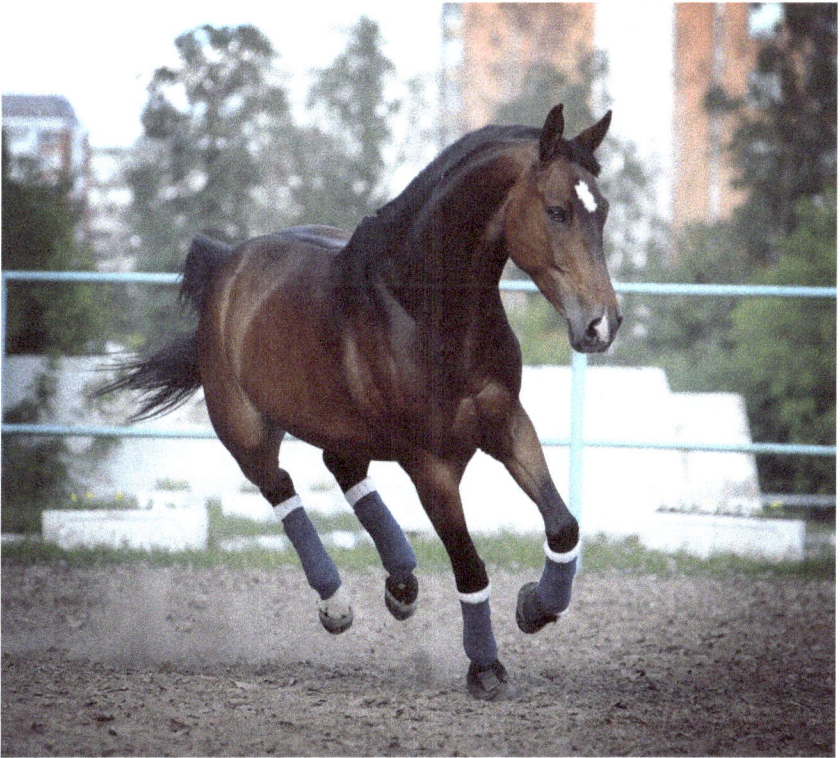

Castration, however is common and recommended for stallions unless you are experienced with stallions or have breeding intentions. Castration is the surgery to remove the testicles. It is also known as gelding.

When a stallion is castrated (gelded), he is then a gelding. The removal of the testicles results in the removal of male hormones. This results in avoiding stallion behavior.

-+

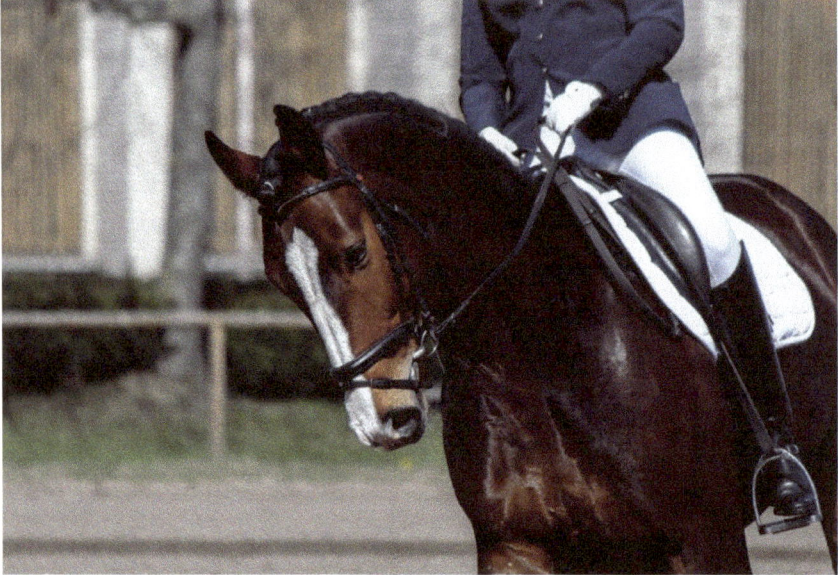

Reasons to castrate include:

- quieter behavior – stallions may be aggressive and unpredictable - even dangerous
- easier to train
- may exercise geldings any time with other horses
- even temperament
- easier housing in barns and pastures
- not having to separate from others -as separating the colts/stallions from the fillies/mares
- avoiding some states' laws requiring special considerations for housing and pasture fencing for stallions

There are several methods a veterinarian may choose from to complete a castration. Ask your veterinarian for their recommendations.

When to Castrate

Some castrate stallions when they are very young- even as young as six months - while some prefer to wait a full year to castrate.

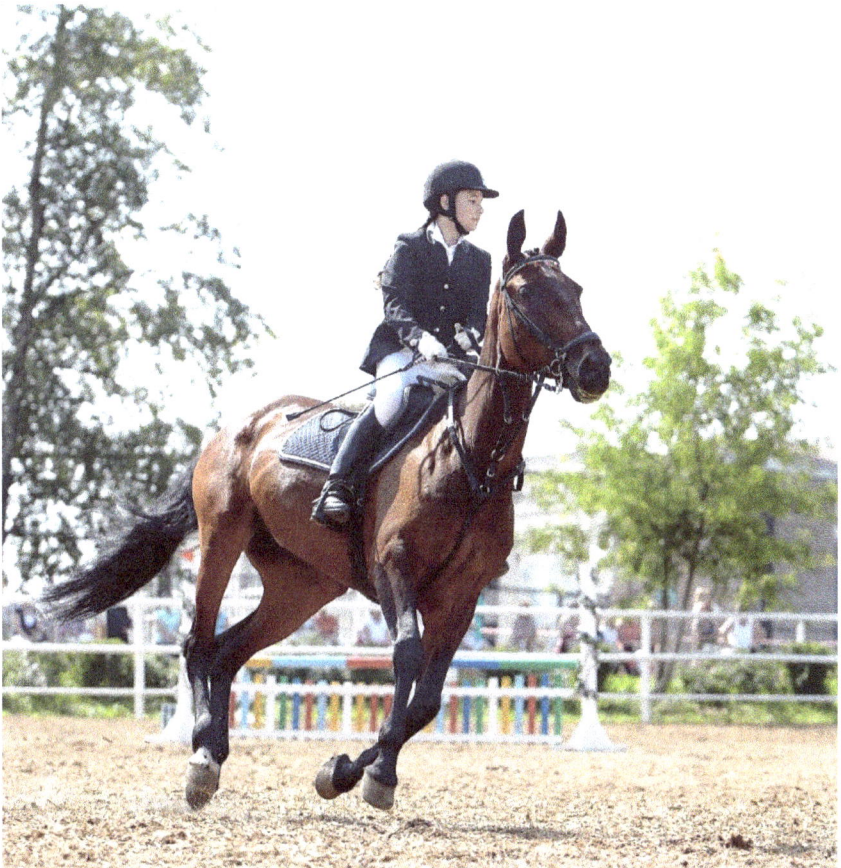

This author feels the younger the stallion is when castrated, the easier the procedure due to older horses having larger testicles and larger blood vessels.

Regarding the time of year, it's generally best to castrate during cool weather if possible so flies aren't as significant an issue to irritate or infect fresh surgical incisions.

Castration Aftercare

After castrating a horse, the veterinarian and owner must monitor the recovering horse closely.

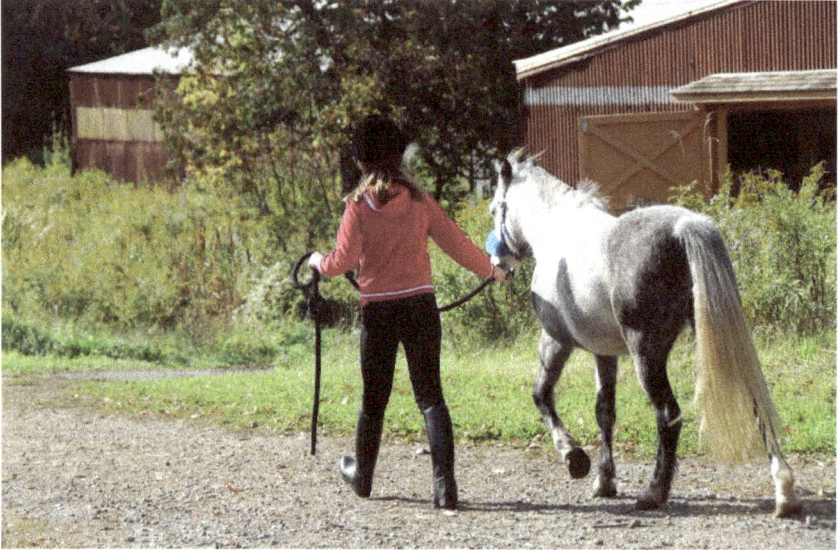

Ask if your veterinarian recommends keeping the horse confined for the first 12 to 24 hours following surgery to make sure the blood clots well in the surgical area.

After this initial period, most veterinarians recommend exercising the horse to prevent excessive swelling and help expel drainage from the incisions.

Ask your veterinarian for his/her recommendations for after castration activity.

Additional Aftercare Considerations

It is not recommended to just turn a horse out on pasture unsupervised after being castrated because when horses are castrated they have pain that may stop them from exercising sufficiently.

Some horses may appear lame (stiff or limping) because of pain when they bring their rear legs forward with swelling to the scrotal area.

The owner should take the horse's temperature daily – if there is a fever, they may need antibiotics. A veterinarian should examine the horse.

Some veterinarians administer anti-inflammatory medications such as flunixin meglumine (Banamine) or phenylbutazone (Bute) for swelling and pain after surgery. Ask your veterinarian for their recommendations.

Always make certain the horses being gelded have tetanus vaccines prior to the procedure.

What Can Go Wrong

One of the most common castration complications is excess bleeding. To help avoid this, one may consider keeping the horse calm and quiet for a brief time before and after surgery.
.

Swelling - normal swelling in the surgical area—starting in the sheath—usually occurs 1-3 days after the initial surgery, however, sometimes excessive swelling occurs.

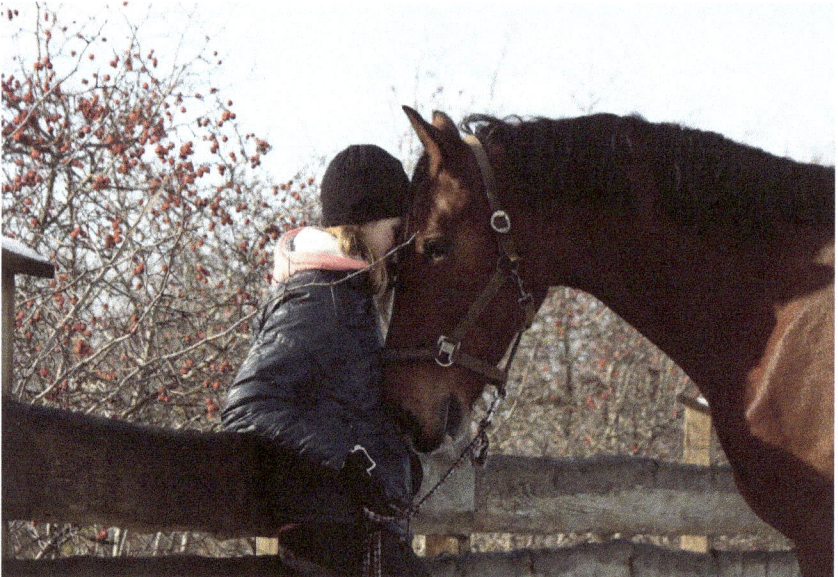

In most cases veterinarians treat excessive groin-area swelling on the farm. Sometimes they do so by:

- reopening the incision site to establish better drainage
- exercising the horse more
- as well as administering anti-inflammatory medication such as banamine or bute

Swelling in the scrotum should be examined daily and closely. If the swelling is excessive, it may indicate

- a hematoma (collection of blood)
- infection
- or a hernia.

A hematoma is a collection of blood in a ball-like shape and is not generally serious.

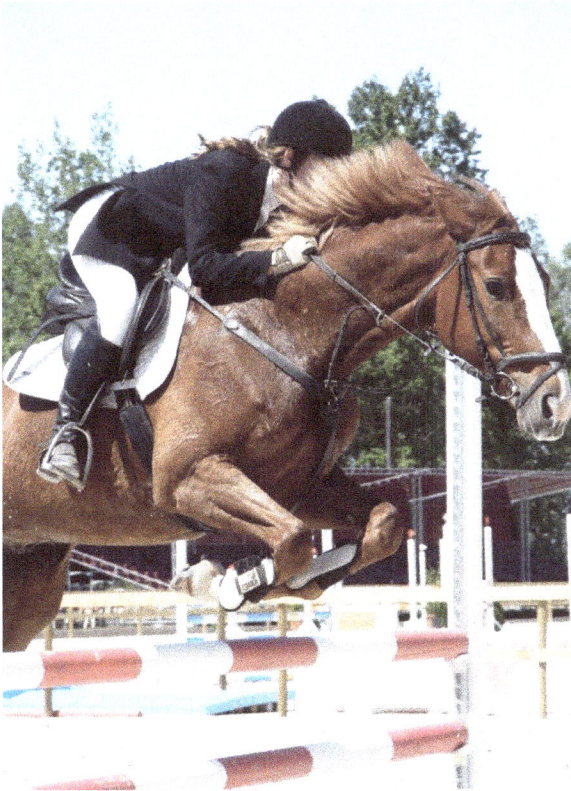

Infection may be detected by fever and loss of appetite.

If infection is present, you should consult your veterinarian so he or she can examine the surgical site and treat as needed.

One of the most serious castration complications is a scrotal hernia. This occurs when the opening above the testicles is larger than normal and allows the small intestine to slip into the scrotal sac.

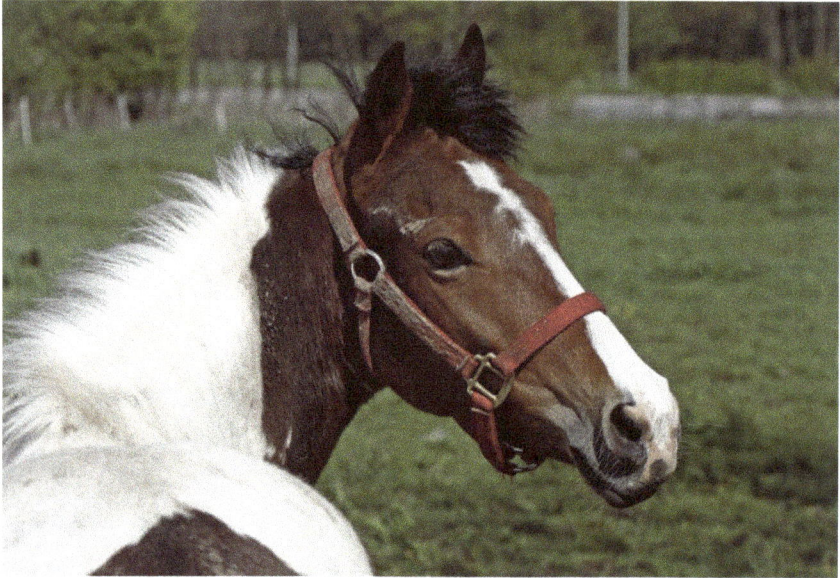

Because this occurs soon following recovery from anesthesia, horses require close observation after the surgery.

Herniation is a surgical emergency and is life threatening. To make certain there is minimal danger of this happening, veterinarians can feel the area in the scrotum above the testicle called the inguinal ring before castrating to make certain it is small and therefore safe to perform a castration.

It is recommended to castrate every horse not intended for breeding.

Chapter 5

What to Expect When Your Mare is Expecting

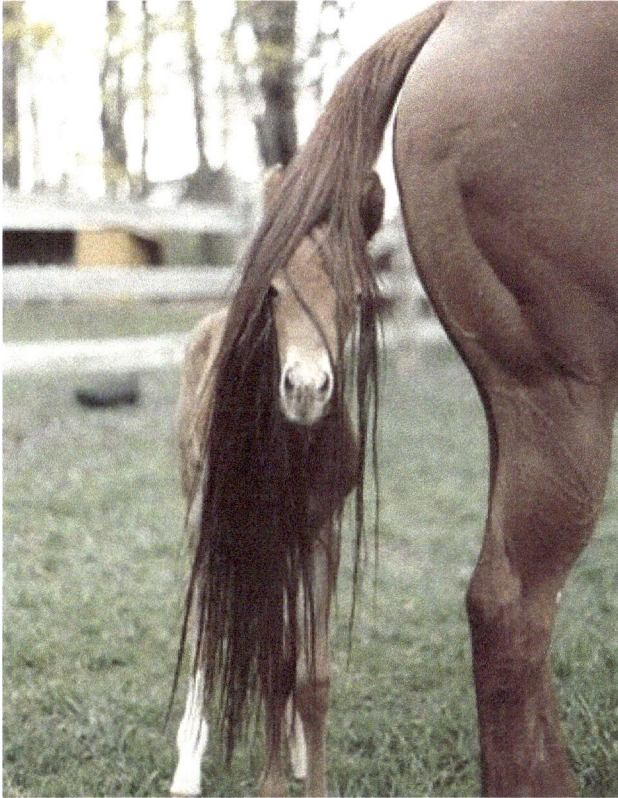

Horse breeding is reproduction in horses and involves the human-directed process of selecting mares and stallions to make desired foals - especially for purebred horses for purposes of racing, jumping, and other uses.

Modern breeding options increase chances of becoming pregnant, having a healthy pregnancy, and successful delivery of foals.

Intentional breeding allows one to predict the time of year the mare will deliver her foal – some breeds prefer certain foaling times.

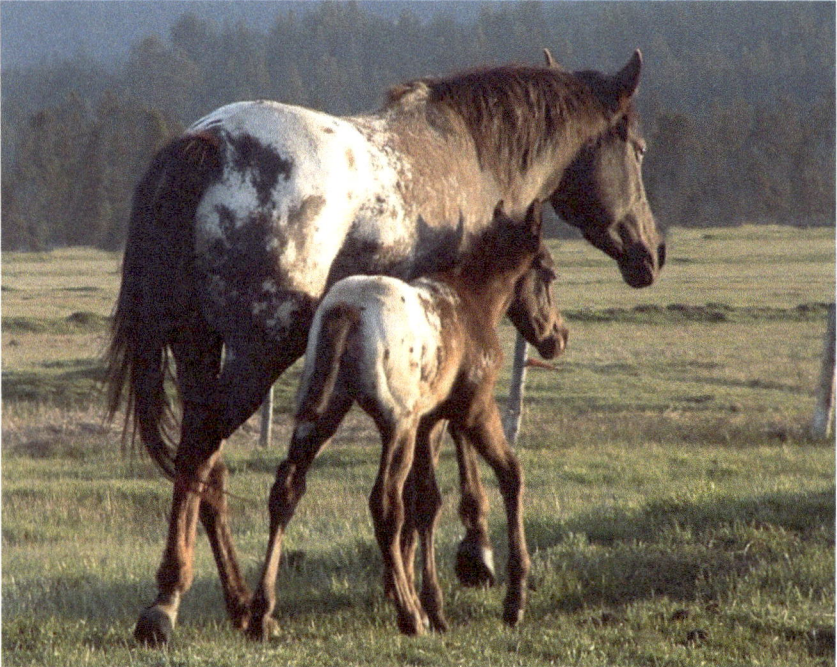

Some common definitions:

- the stallion- the male horse- known as the sire
- the mare-the female- known as the dam
- the foal – the offspring of the mare and sire
- colt- a male foal
- filly- a female foal
- breeding – causing pregnancy in a female horse

Getting Pregnant

- estrous –mares cycle every 19-22 days with the average being 21 days – this is the time they are receptive to the stallion
- make certain the mare is healthy and able to be bred
- pregnancy lasts 11 months – about 335-340 days
- ultrasound may be performed at 19-21 days – this is advantageous because if the mare is not pregnant, it is possible to rebreed her on the next cycle – sooner than can be determined by physical palpation of the mare at 35 days
- palpation- is manually feeling the uterus for pregnancy and is completed at 35, 60, and 90 days- size and presence of the foal is determined- after 60 days, the uterus extends over the pelvic brim and cannot be felt until late in pregnancy when the foal is large and moving and easily felt
- udder development is usually obvious by 2-5 weeks before delivery

Methods of breeding include:

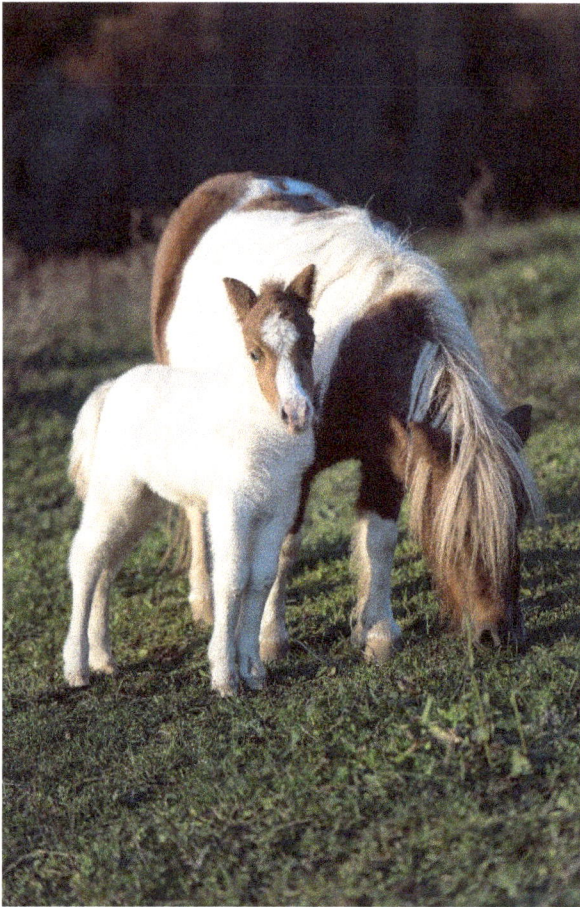

- natural service – AKA live cover- is where a stallion physically breeds the mare
- artificial insemination – where semen is collected from the stallion and instilled into the uterus of the mare by a trained person
- embryo transfer – where 2 mares are hormonally synchronized for pregnancy, one mare is bred and her fertilized embryos are flushed from her uterus then instilled into another mare to be the surrogate mother horse for the foal

Natural Service/Live cover

This is when the mare is bred by the stallion.

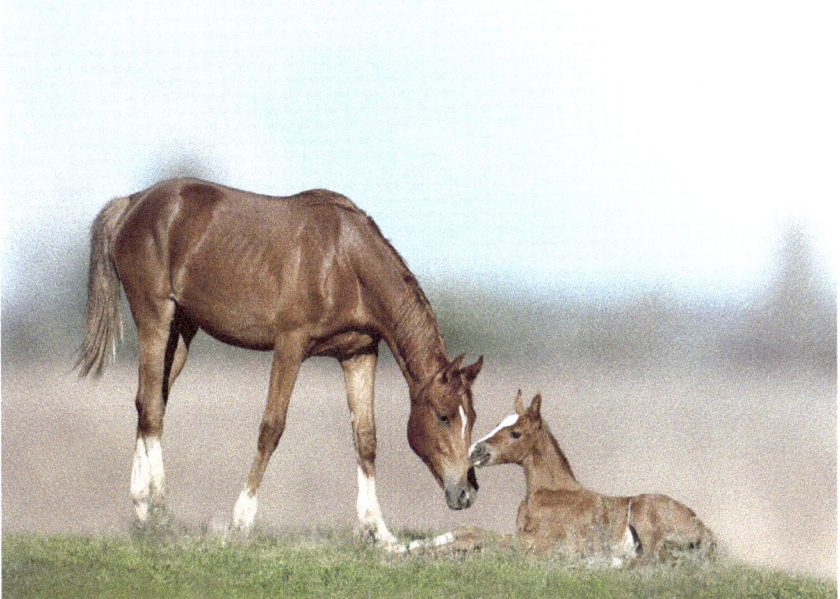

The mare is brought to the stallion's residence and bred when she is receptive to him. This is preferred because one can insure breeding has been accomplished and there is less chance of injury. Mares may kick and injure stallions trying to breed them. Hobbling the back legs may be considered if the mare tries to kick the stallion. This is an important safety concern, especially if the breed requires natural service- such as Thoroughbred horses.

Some choose to turn mares out in a pasture with the stallion for several days to breed naturally. This is risky and may result in injury or the mare not being bred.

Preparing to Breed

Teasing- is when the mare is presented to the stallion. Most breeders walk the mare past the stallion. If she is receptive – she typically stands, raises her tail, and/or urinates and he reacts to her. This indicates she is ready to be bred.

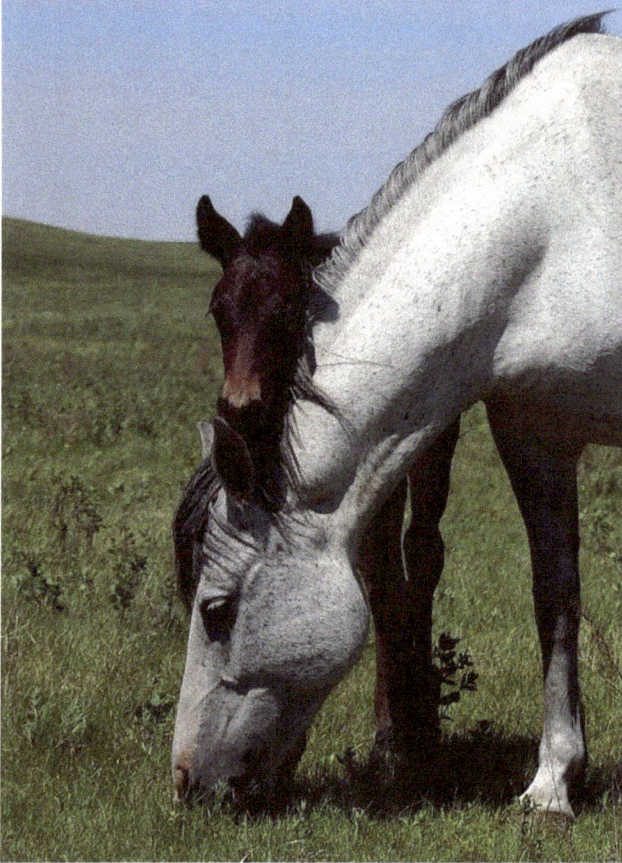

When the mare is ready, both the mare and stallion should be cleaned.

It is safest to have someone hold the mare while one or more handlers handle the stallion. When two handlers are present, one can be on each side of the stallion- controlling the situation to prevent injury to the horses or handlers.

Artificial Insemination (AI)

Artificial insemination-is when semen is collected from the stallion and instilled into the mare when she is ready to become pregnant.

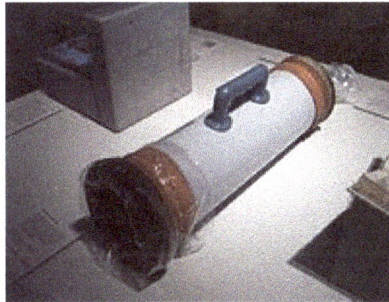

An artificial vagina- pictured above- is used to collect the semen.

The stallion is trained to mount a 'dummy' mare on the farm or a live mare may be used initially and then removed as the semen collection is completed.

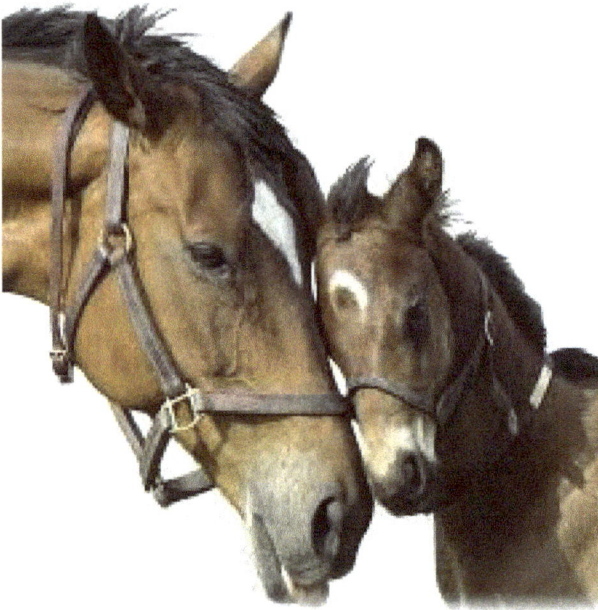

The semen may be:
- fresh- collected and immediately placed into a mare that is on the same farm
- cooled- and shipped to another farm to be placed into a receptive mare
- frozen for future use in mares

The semen is instilled with a pipette after the mare is cleaned.

Advantages to Artificial insemination

Artificial insemination (AI) has several advantages over live cover and has a very similar conception rate:

- since the mare and stallion do not have contact, breeding accidents are minimized or eliminated
- AI allows international breeding because semen may be shipped across continents to mares that would not be able to breed to a particular stallion otherwise
- a mare does not have to travel to the stallion – this makes the process less stressful for her and, if she already has a foal, the foal does not have to travel
- AI allows more than one mare to be bred from one stallion collection because the semen may be divided and used in several mares
- AI reduces the chance of spreading sexually transmitted diseases between mares and stallions
- AI allows mares or stallions with health issues, such as sore legs or backs to be bred without discomfort- and allows the stallion and /or the mare to continue to breed
- frozen semen may be stored for a long time and used to breed mares even after the stallion is no longer alive – this allows his lines to continue - however, sometimes the semen of some stallions does not freeze well or some breed registries may not permit the registration of foals resulting from the use of frozen semen after a stallion's death

Embryo Transfer

Embryo transfer –is when 2 mares are hormonally synchronized for pregnancy. One mare (the donor mare) is bred and her ….

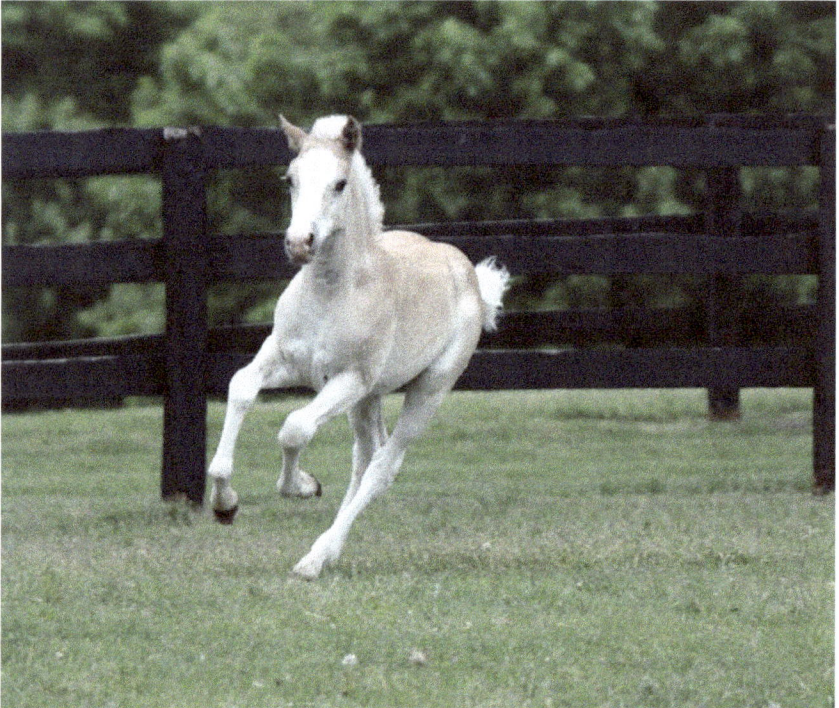

….. fertilized embryos are flushed from her uterus a few days after insemination and instilled into a second mare (the recipient mare) intended to be the surrogate mother horse for the foal.

Advantages of embryo transfer include:

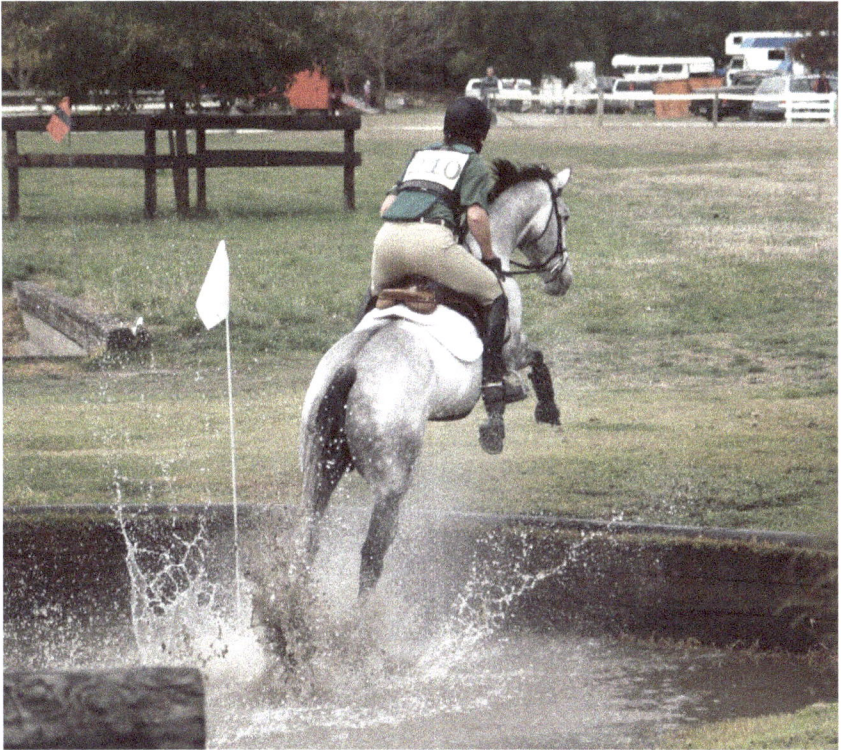

- the donor mare can continue being ridden and used for the purpose she is valuable- jumping, dressage, racing, eventing, etc - and still reproduce a valuable foal with her genetic make- up
- sometimes older mares are not able to maintain a pregnancy and embryo transfer allows a younger mare to carry the pregnancy
- the donor mare may have health issues or be painful and unable to maintain a pregnancy
- more than one foal can be reproduced in a year with embryo transfer- this is an advantage especially if the foals are valuable

Care of the pregnant mare

Some general care guidelines include:

- mares should receive specific nutrition to ensure that they and their foals are healthy - ask your veterinarian for their recommendations for feeding your pregnant mare
- mares should be given vaccinations against diseases such as the rhinopneumonitis (EHV-1) virus (which can cause abortions) as well as vaccines for other major diseases that may occur in a given region of the world including tetanus and rabies
- pre-foaling vaccines are recommended 4–6 weeks prior to foaling - this maximizes the protective antibodies discussed in chapter 2 in the mare's colostrum
- most veterinarians recommend mares be dewormed a few weeks prior to delivery of the foal
- mares may be exercised - used for riding or driving during most of their pregnancy – but should be moderated when a mare is heavily in foal
- exercise may be contraindicated in areas with high or low ambient temperatures

Foaling

Preparing for the foal includes:

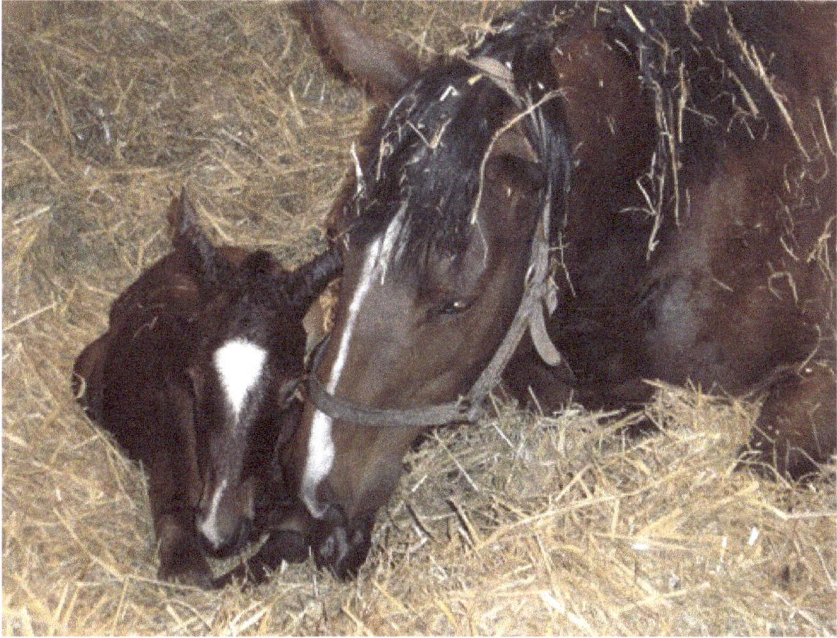

- a foaling stall that is large and clutter free – this allows close monitoring of the foal and mare and protects them from harsh weather in many climates
- STRAW bedding is preferred over wood shavings
- smaller breeders sometimes use a small fenced pen with a large shed for foaling, or they may remove a wall between two box stalls in a small barn to make a large stall
- in milder climates, mares may foal outside - often in paddocks built specifically for foaling - especially on larger farms – however, this may result in larger losses of mares and foals because there is little monitoring

(Continued) Preparing for the foal:

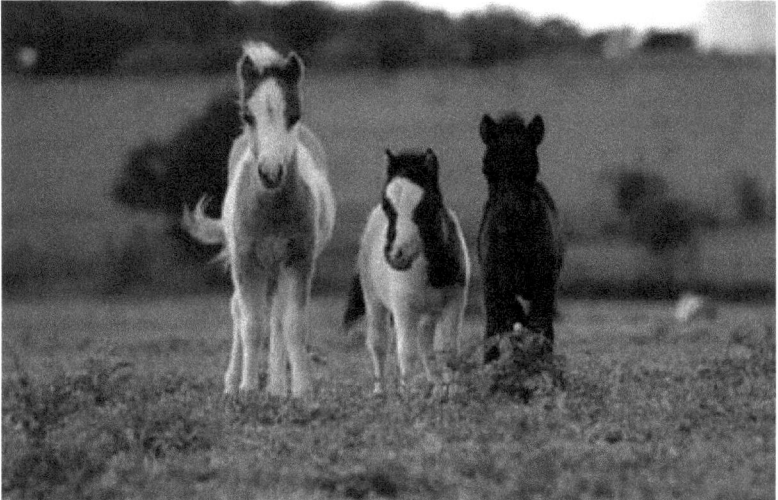

- many farms use cameras or monitors to alert human managers when the mare is about to foal
- some farms have care takers who watch the mares directly for signs of and actual foaling when they are close to having their foals – this is to help when needed
- most mares have their foals at night or early in the morning, and prefer to give birth alone
- mares close to foaling are usually separated from other horses - both for the benefit of the mare and the safety of the soon-to-be-delivered foal

Delivering the Foal

Labor is rapid in the horse- often no more than 30 minutes.

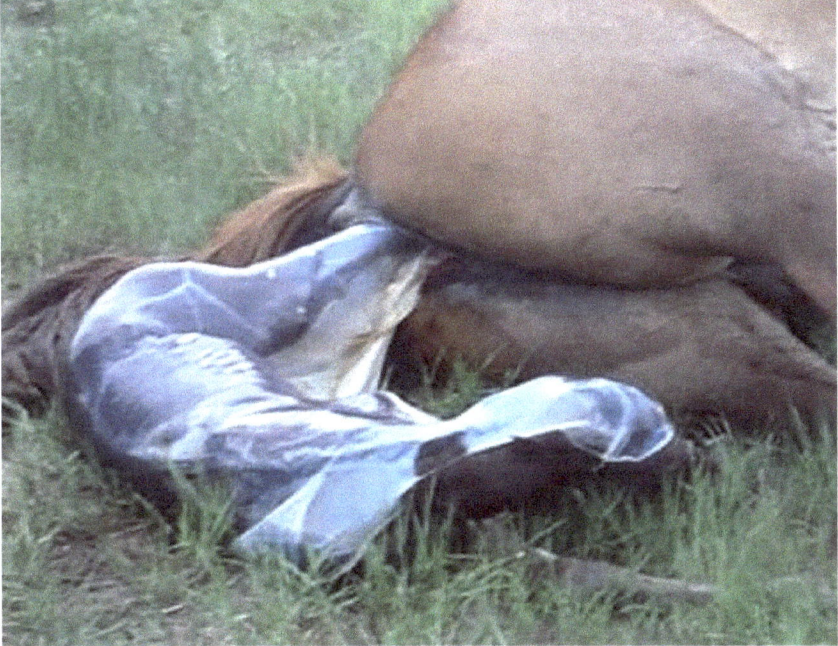

From the time the feet of the foal appear to full delivery is often only about 15 to 20 minutes.

The mare expels a watery fluid- the amniotic fluid around the foal.

Then the foal arrives with both front feet and the nose between them.

After the foal is born, the mare will lick the newborn foal to clean it and help blood circulation.

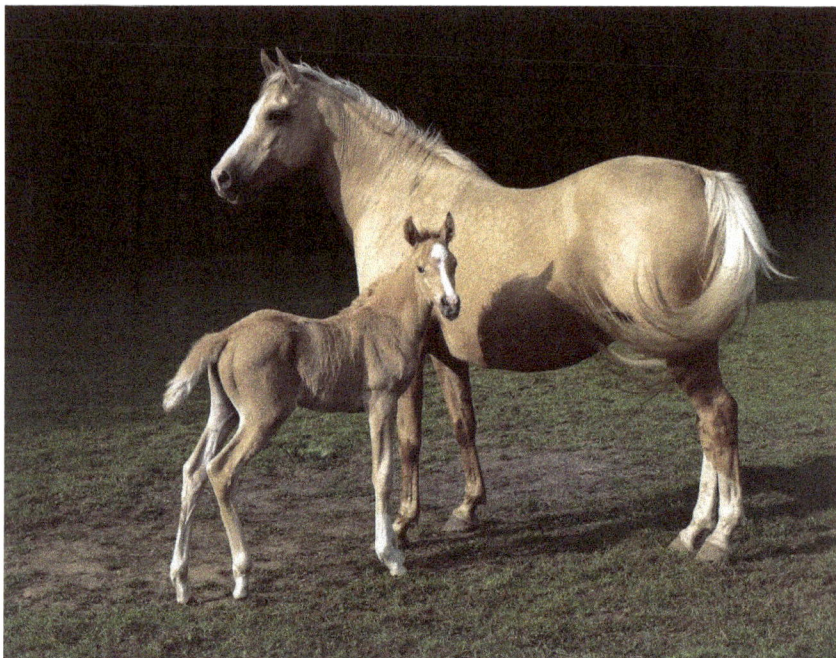

A foal should stand and nurse within the first hour of life.

To create a bond with her foal, the mare licks and nuzzles the foal, enabling her to distinguish the foal from others.

Some mares are aggressive when protecting their foals, and may attack other horses or unfamiliar humans that come near their newborns. Be careful.

The placenta should pass within 2-3 hours after delivery- it should be examined to make certain it is all present. Retained tissues is cause for concern because this can lead to uterine infection and infertility or founder (laminitis) if untreated or unattended to. This may also lead to loss of the mare.

FOAL CARE

It is critical that the newborn stands and nurses soon after birth.

The first milk is a special milk- called colostrum. Colostrum contains the proteins which protect the foal from the major diseases of horses.

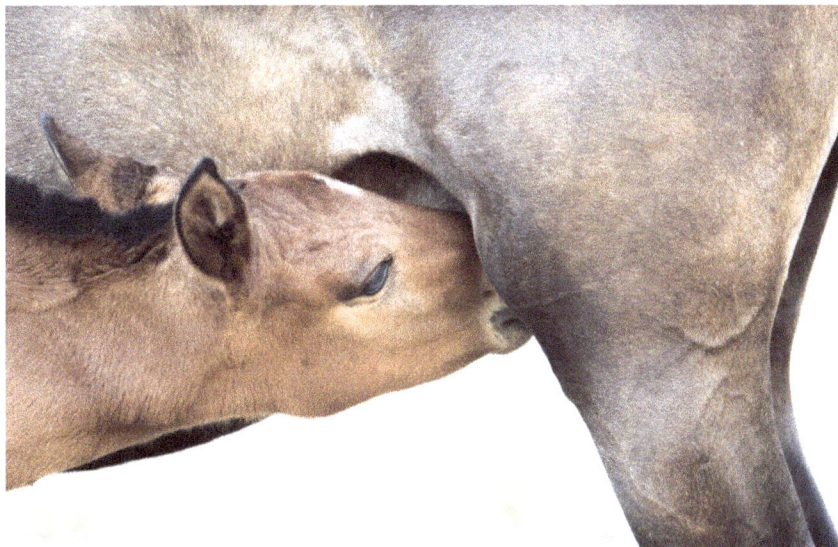

The foal's intestines are only able to absorb the large protective proteins for about 24 hours, however, the foal usually nurses and obtains these necessary proteins in the first 12 hours after being born. Peak absorption occurs during the first 6-12 hours following birth. This process is called 'passive transfer' of the mother's protection for disease to the foal.

As mentioned, vaccinating mares prior to delivery allows greater amounts of protective antibodies in her colostrum.

Sometimes the mare's udder distends with milk/colostrum and is sensitive to the point she refuses to allow the foal to nurse or is a first-time mother and doesn't know how.

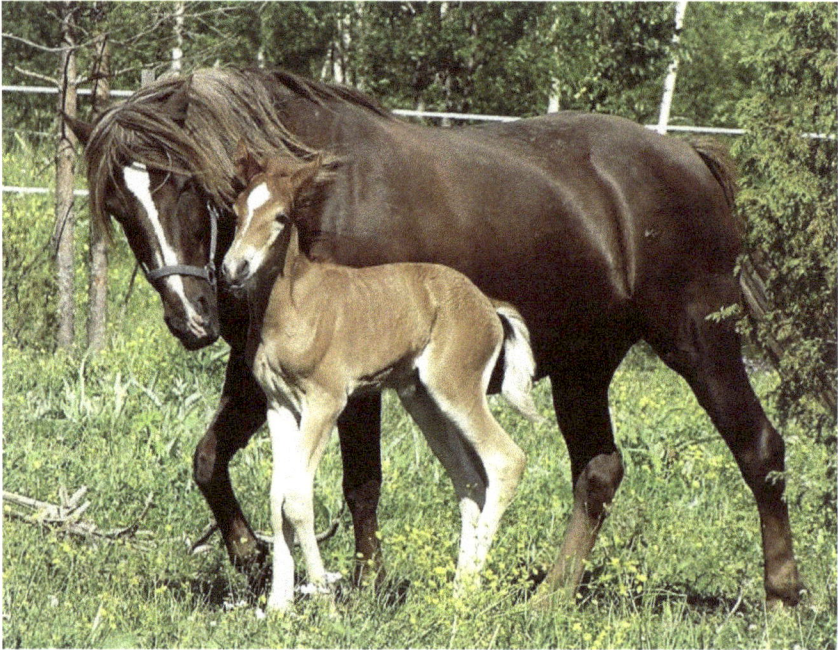

These mares need to be 'milked' manually to obtain the colostrum.

The colostrum can be placed in a bowl and offered to the foal- they will suck it up. If the foal does not drink the colostrum, a tube can be passed to administer mother's colostrum.

Colostrum replacement is also available.

Colostrum and passive transfer of antibodies against disease are critical to the health of the foal. If passive transfer does not occur, veterinary care is important to ensure survival of the foal. The foal may require plasma administered intravenously to provide the missing or deficient protective antibodies. This is also critical if the mare is lost for any reason in delivering the foal.

It is recommended to test the foal for 'passive transfer' of the protective proteins from the mother. A veterinarian can perform this test.

Protective proteins in colostrum are called IgG. Healthy foals that have nursed and absorbed adequate colostrum have an IgG concentration in their bloodstream of at least 800 mg/dl.

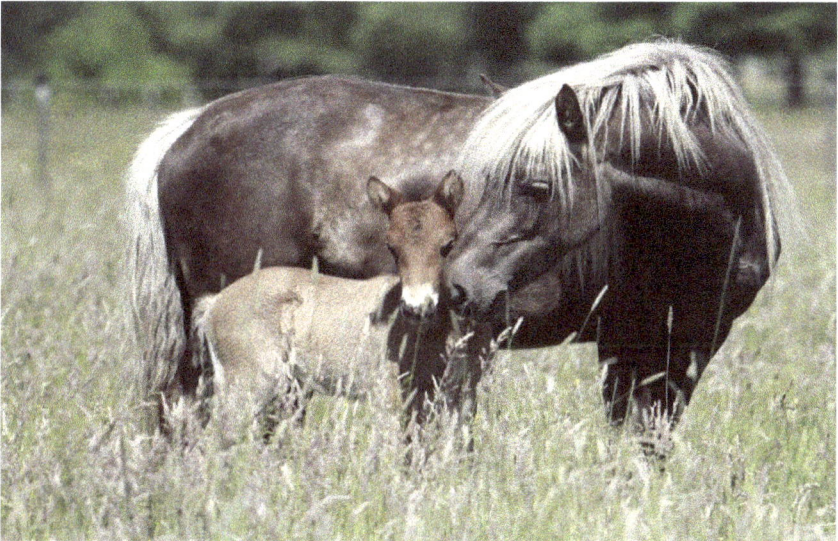

A veterinarian can draw a blood sample from a foal within 12-18 hours of delivery and can quickly and accurately measure the IgG concentration.

Newborn foals with IgG concentrations less than 400 mg/dl should receive supplemental colostrum and/or a plasma transfusion to provide vital antibodies that help reduce the risk of serious bacterial and viral infections during the first few months of life.

Foals should be examined within 24 hours after delivery.

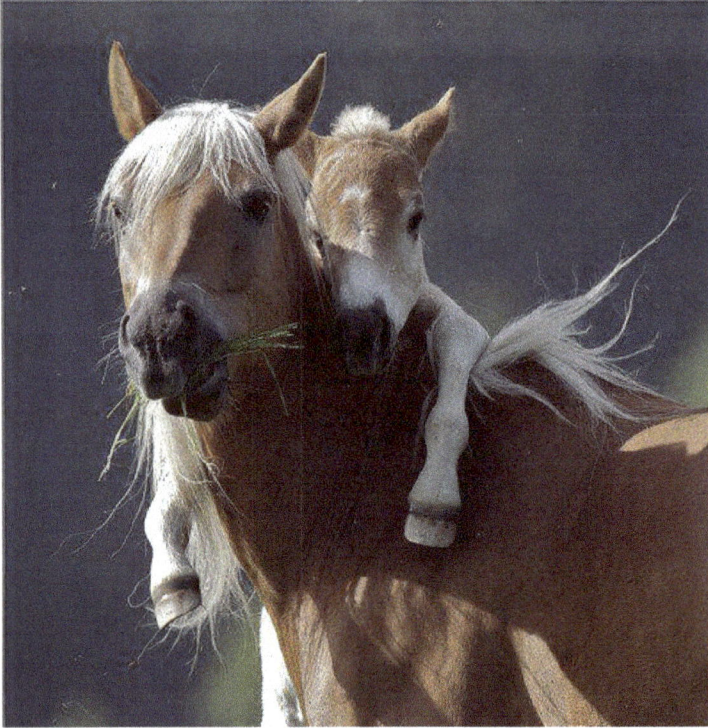

Many owners place antiseptic mediation onto a foal's navel to prevent infection - some dip the foal's umbilical stump with dilute chlorhexidine or iodine twice daily for 2-3 days or until the stump is dry.

Another important part of foal care is to make certain the foal passes the first manure- called meconium. Foals typically pass this within 12-24 hours.

Meconium does not look like usual horse manure – it is pasty or pelleted in consistency and dark brown or black.

If the meconium does not pass naturally, an enema is given to prevent impaction.

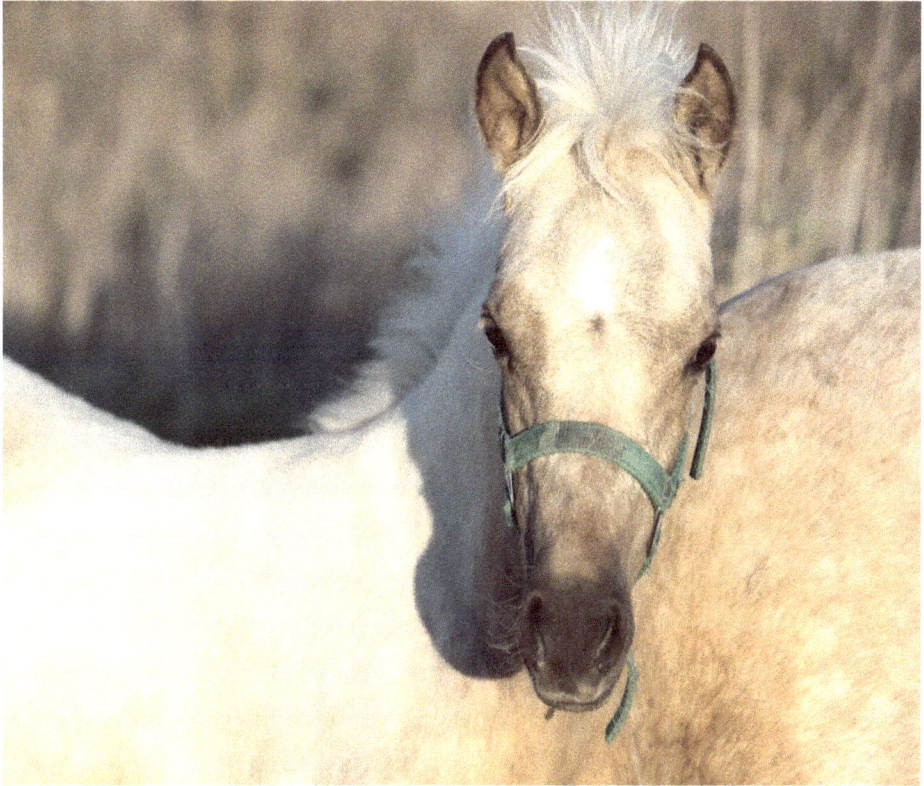

Newborn foals should be observed frequently during the first few weeks of life.

It is important to detect signs of disease early.

Often the first signs of a sick foal is weakness and decreased nursing vigor- which may be noticed by distention and pain to the mother's udder.

Young foals are at risk for a variety of respiratory diseases and diarrhea. Always monitor a young foal's breathing rate and effort, body temperature, nursing behavior and manure consistency.

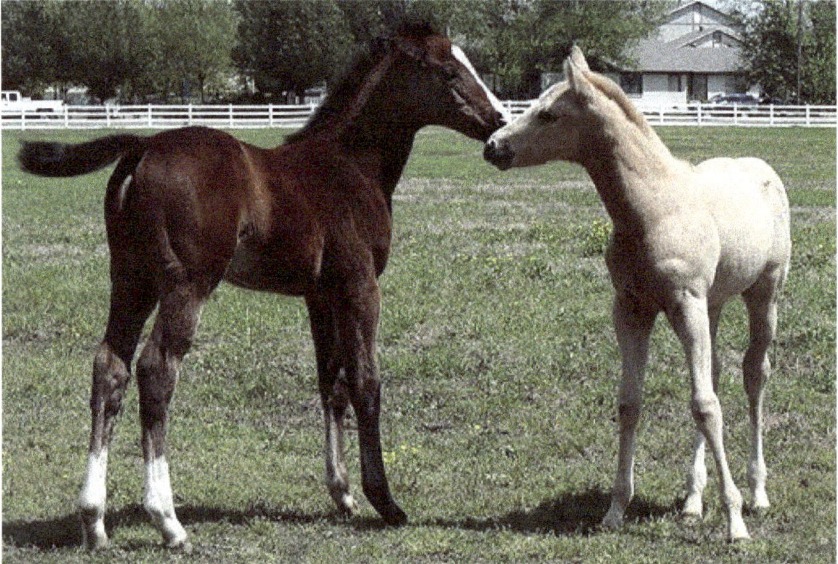

The protective proteins- the antibodies foals receive when they first nurse eventually decline. To continue to protect for foals, they need to be vaccinated.

Timing of the vaccinations is critical. When mother's colostrum derived antibodies are present, the foal's body thinks it is protected and will not make antibodies of their own when vaccinated.

Since mom's protection is temporary protection, vaccines need to be given when they are no longer protecting the foal.

The timing of the vaccines is determined by whether the foal suckled well or not well when born.

Ask your veterinarian for foal vaccine recommendations

When to Worry

Most horse births happen without complications; however, significant complications may occur.

Many owners have first aid supplies on hand and a veterinarian on call in case of a birthing emergency.

The most important thing to remember is that if there are any difficulties, a veterinarian should be called immediately. Horse births are generally fast and problems escalate quickly. Mares and foals may be lost if assistance is not sought quickly.

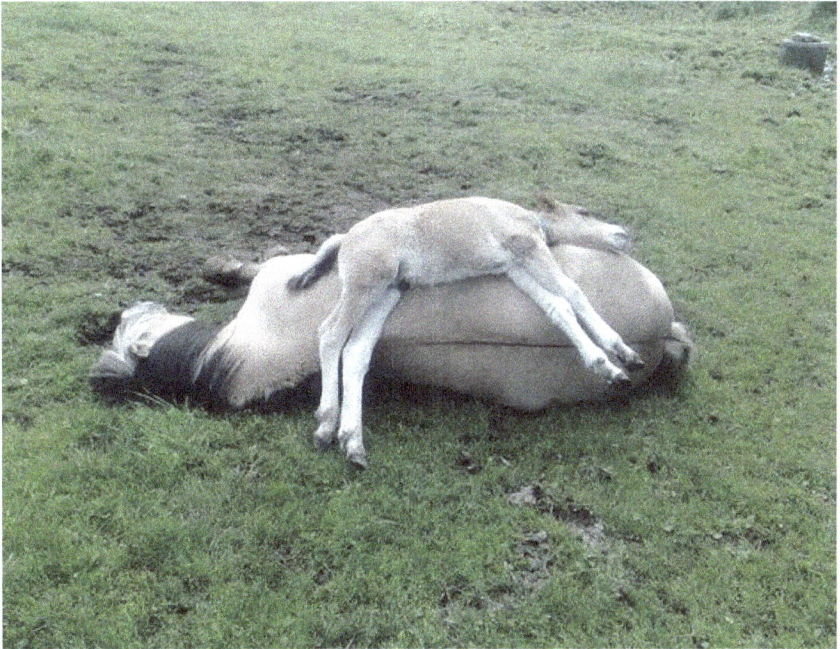

Dystocia is defined as difficulty delivering the foal. The most common reason for dystocia is a foal in the wrong position for birth.

Foal patrol helps determine difficulties early.

One must know the difference from the front and back feet, breach births are not recommended for horses.

Caretakers supervising foaling should also watch the mare to be sure she passes the placenta in a timely fashion, and that it is complete with no fragments remaining in the uterus, where retained fetal membranes could cause a serious inflammatory condition called endometritis and/or infection.

If the placenta is not removed from the stall after it is passed, a mare will often eat it - an instinct from the wild, where blood would attract predators.

Foals develop rapidly, and within a few hours a foal can travel with the herd.

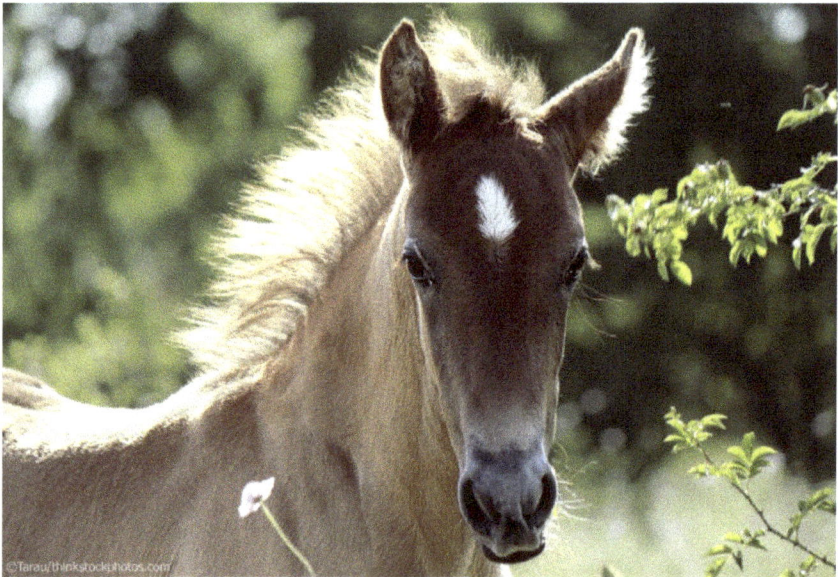

In domestic breeding, the foal and dam are usually separated from the herd for a while, but within a few weeks are typically pastured with the other horses.

Foals begin to eat hay, grass and grain alongside the mare at about 4 weeks old. By 10–12 weeks foals typically require more nutrition than the mare's milk can supply. Foal feeders are available to introduce grain to growing foals to prevent their moms from eating their ration.

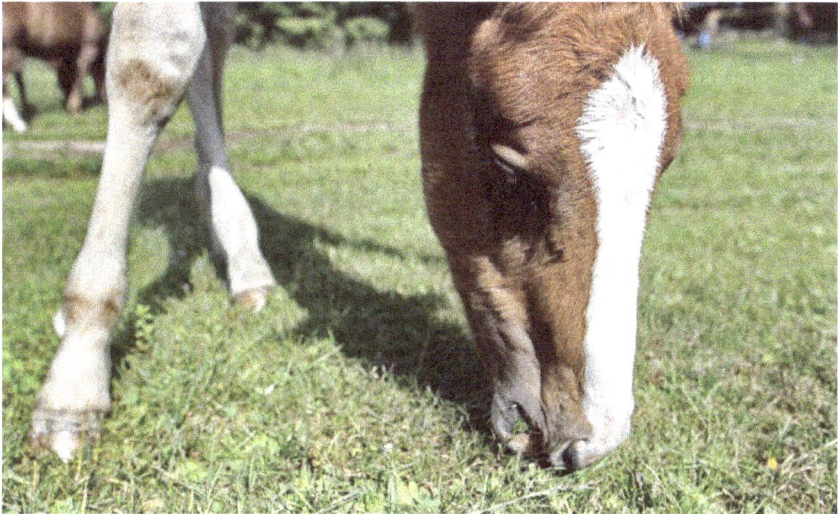

Foals are typically weaned at 4–8 months of age.

There are several ways to wean a foal. Ask your veterinarian for recommendations for safe weaning.

FOAL PROOF THE PASTURE

Fencing and footing are important parts of foal safety.

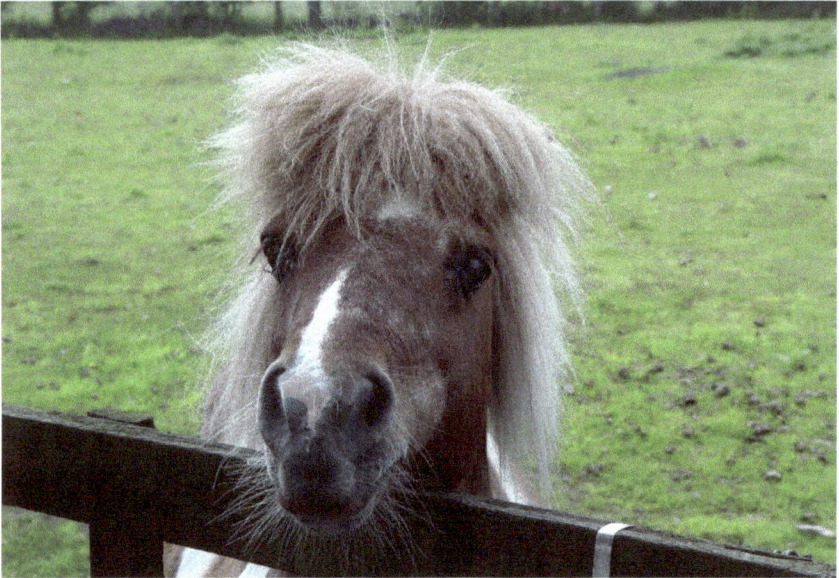

Make certain there are no sharp edges- barbed wire is not recommended for horses or foals.

Make certain there are no gaps in the fencing.

4-5 feet tall fencing is recommended – decide based on the size of the horses in the pasture areas.

Provide a source of water always.

Make certain there are no holes in the pasture ground that may cause injury to the mares and foals.

Make certain the pasture is accessible to you.

Chapter 6

Dental care

Dentition

Healthy teeth are important for the overall health of the horse.

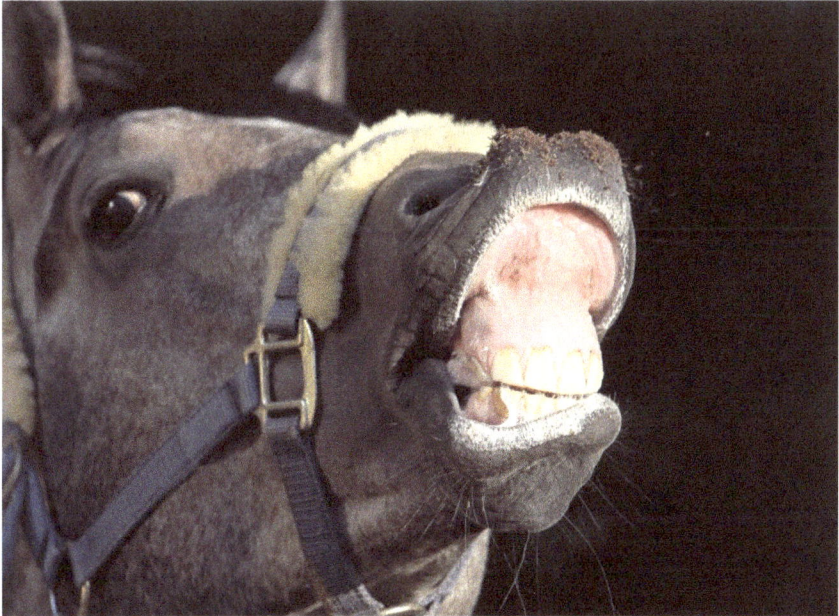

Poor dentition interferes with food breakdown and usage.

Proper and routine care of the horse's mouth helps the horse maximize nutrients from the food he or she is eating.

Horses' Teeth

The first deciduous teeth (AKA baby teeth) are also called 'caps' and usually erupt before the foal is born. These are temporary teeth that will 'fall out' or peel away as the adult- permanent teeth grow. Baby teeth are white and milky looking.

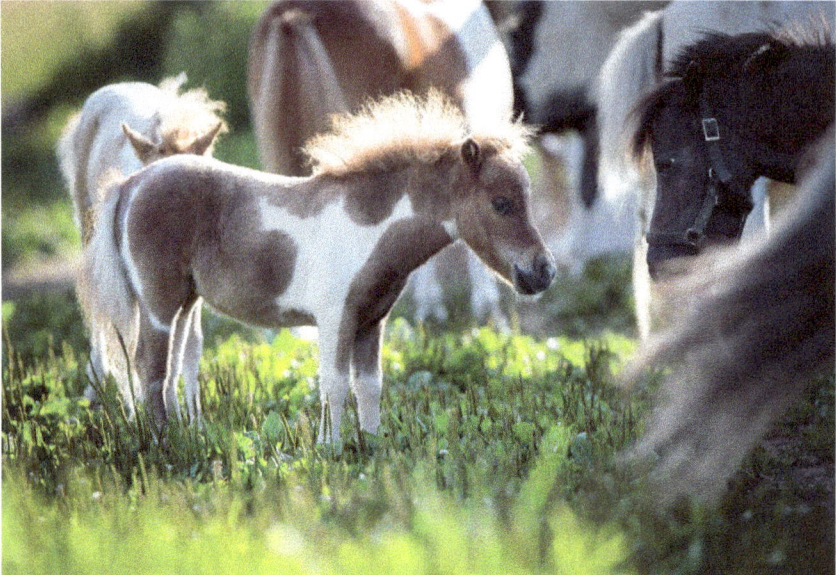

The last deciduous - 'baby teeth' – erupt at about 8 months of age.

Baby teeth start being replaced by adult teeth by 3 years of age.

By 5 years of age, most horses have all their permanent teeth.

Permanent teeth are yellow and brown in color. They are larger in shape.

Aging Horses by Their Teeth

The incisors are the 'front teeth.'

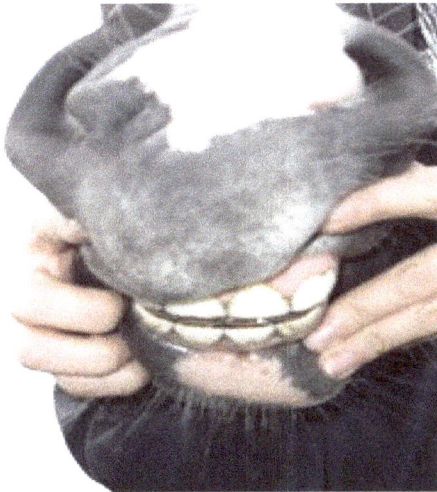

Within days of birth – or at birth- the front incisors come first.

By 9 months of age- all the deciduous – baby, temporary- teeth are present.

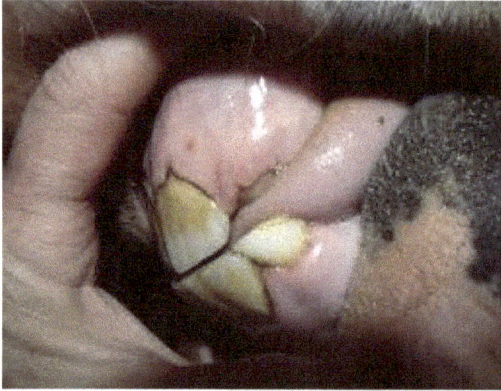

By 12 months of age- the outer incisors are coming in, but are shorter than the other incisors and do not touch.

By 2 years of age- all the incisors are present and their surfaces meet each other.

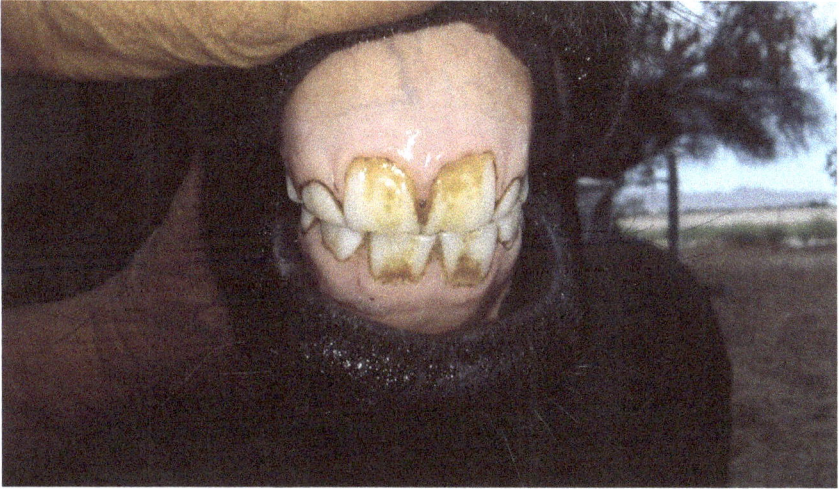

By 3 years of age – the temporary (caps) front two incisors are lost and replaced by the permanent adult teeth.

By 4 years of age - the next two temporary (baby) incisors - the second or middle incisors - are lost and replaced by the permanent adult teeth.

By 5 years of age – the outer temporary incisors are lost and replaced by the permanent adult teeth.
All the incisors are 'adult' incisors by 5 years of age.

After 5 years of age, it becomes more challenging to accurately age horses by their teeth. Purebred horses have registration papers to document the ages of horses, however, many are sold without these papers.

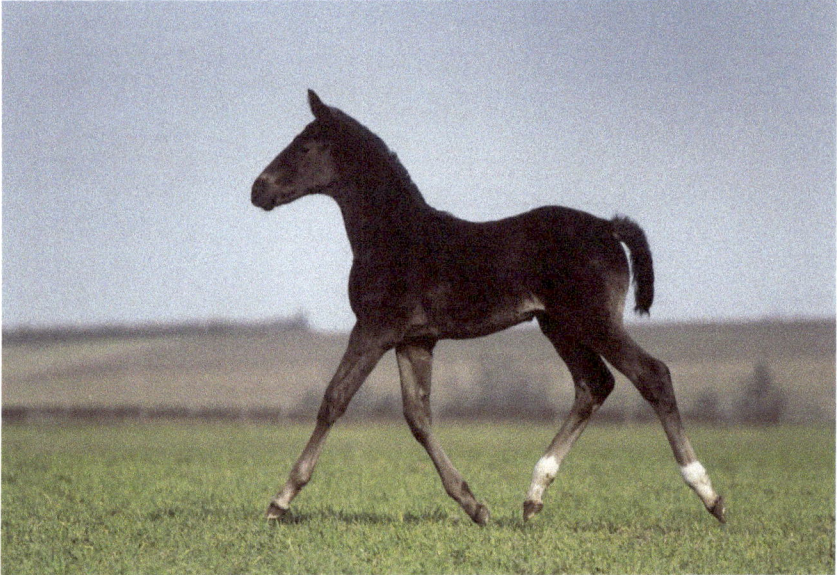

Several other issues must be taken into consideration when aging horses. The teeth are altered by:

- harmful habits such as chewing or cribbing
- poor dental care during the horse's lifetime
- genetics and anatomic defects such as an overbite
- the type of diet fed the horse- for example soft alfalfa hay is less abrasive than some harsher pastures which may even have sand as a base

Some Helpful Hints for Aging Older Horses

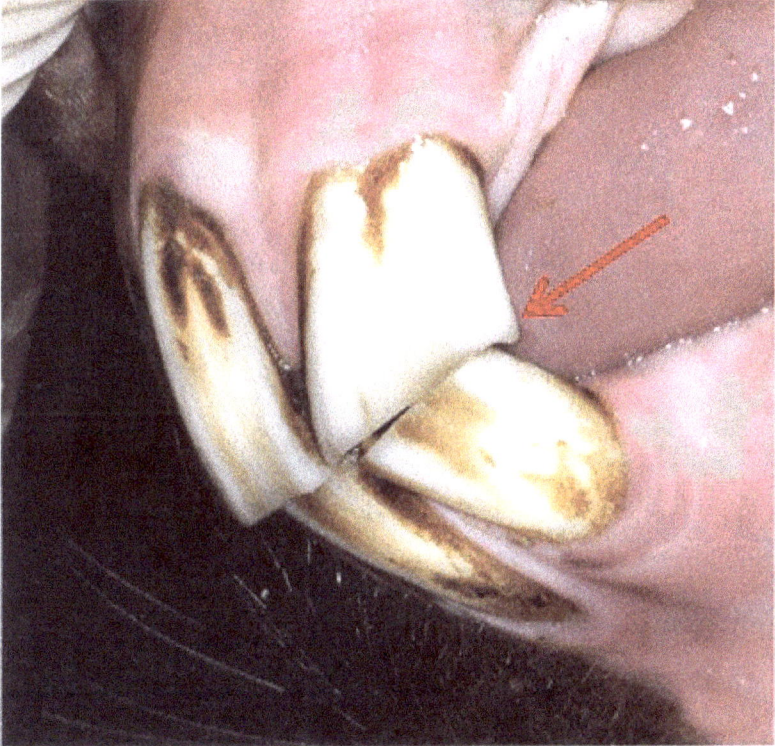

The '7-year hook' – is a hook found on the 'outer' incisor.

Also, associated with the outer incisor, is Galvayne's groove.

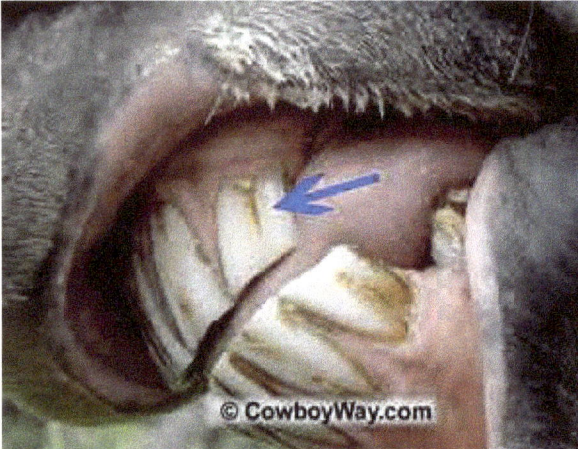

© CowboyWay.com

Galvayne's groove begins to develop on this incisor at about 10 years of age.

The groove extends about half way down the tooth by about 15 years of age.

The groove extends all the way down the length of the tooth by 20 years of age.

The groove begins to disappear on the top half of the tooth by 25 years of age.

The groove disappears completely from this incisor by 30 years of age.

Wolf Teeth

The area between the incisors and molars is called the diastema. This is where the bit sits in the horse's mouth.

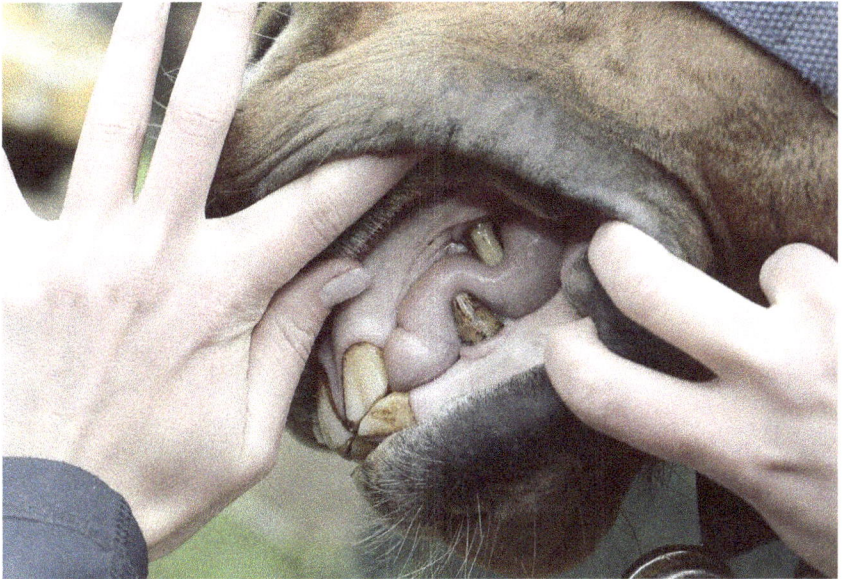

Wolf teeth are small upper premolar teeth that erupt at about 5-12 months of age in about 70% of horses.

These teeth are removed because they can cause discomfort when the bit is introduced in training and riding horses.

Dental Care

Horses chew in a circular motion from one side of their mouth to the other. This motion wears away the horse's teeth and leads to...

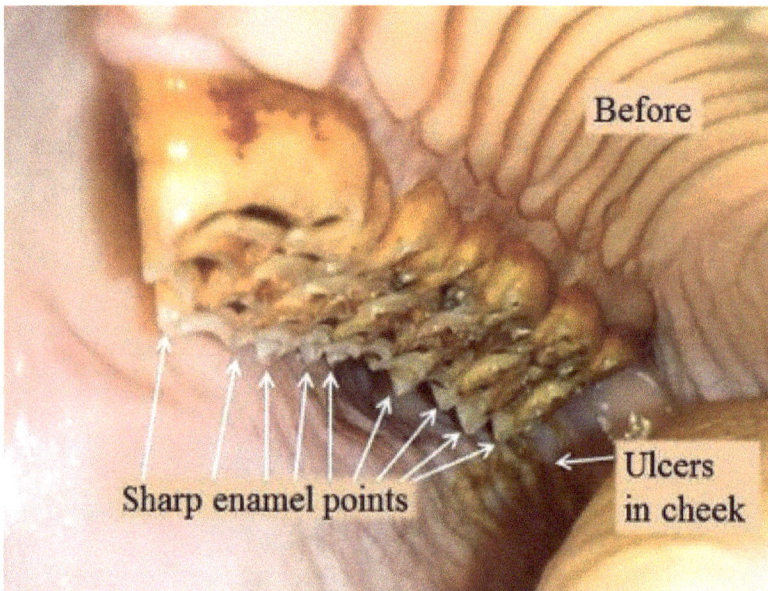

Before

Sharp enamel points

Ulcers in cheek

... the development of sharp points on the outside of the horse's upper molars and on the inside of the horse's lower molars.

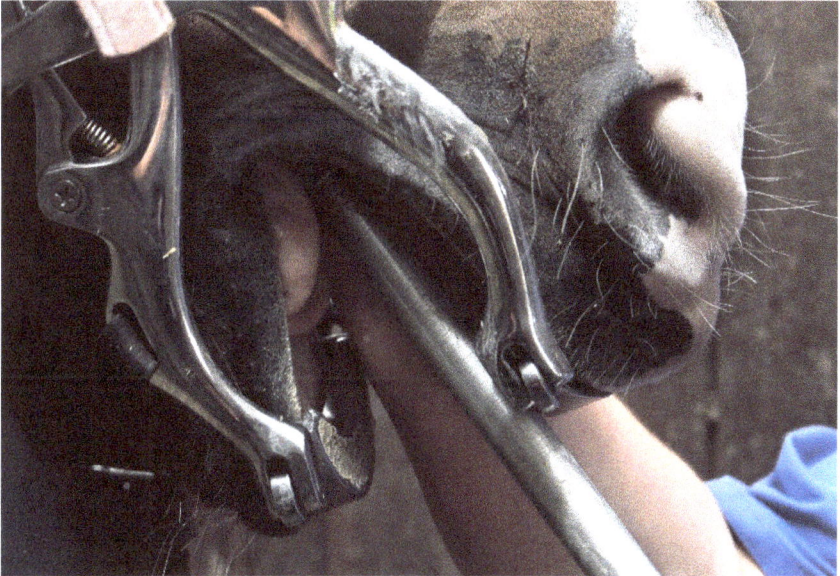

These sharp points must be filed down by floating (filing) the horse's teeth regularly. One to two times per year is recommended.

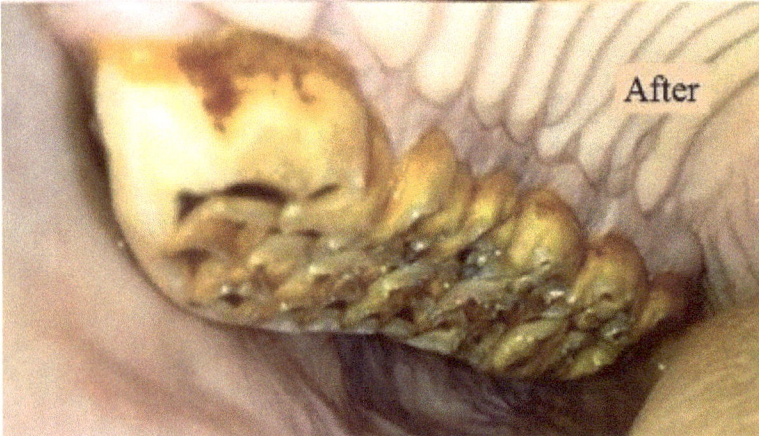

After

Floating, or keeping the horse's teeth filed down, improves the horse's chewing ability and allow him to better digest foods that he or she is eating.

SPECIAL NEEDS FOR OLDER HORSES

As a horse chews, develops sharp edges, and has these filed, over the years, eventually the teeth come to the end of their ability to push down though the bones of the jaw - this means they 'run out of teeth' and eventually the teeth are lost.

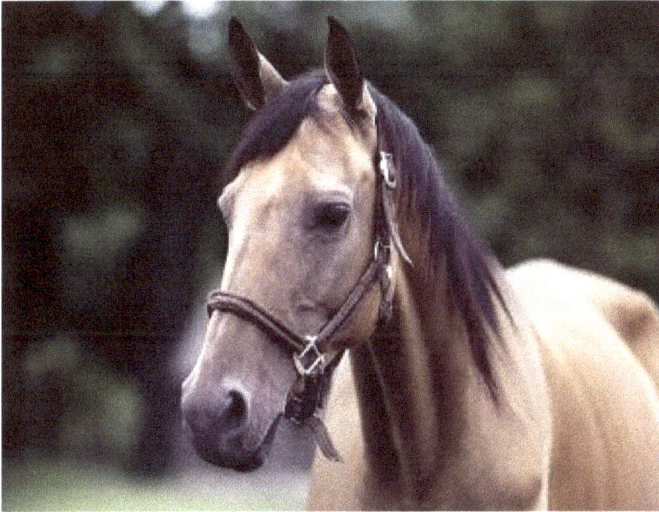

This process continues throughout the life of the horse, but by the time the horse approaches his or her 30s, most of the tooth may be worn down to the roots. This leaves the older horse with little ability to chew and digest foods he or she would ordinarily eat.

Older horses may need to be fed alternative feed.

Many feed companies make senior horse feeds that is softer in texture than ordinary horse feeds-making chewing easier.

Pelleted foods are also available. These feeds are helpful because the horse only needs to swallow the feed to receive the nutrition.

Concentrates fed in the form of pelleted feed can be wet down and softened to make a gruel that is easy for the horse to chew as well.

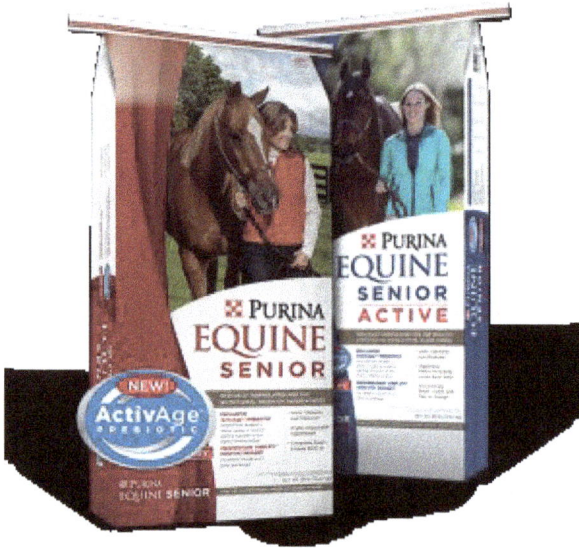

Nutritional needs of aging horses will vary greatly between individuals.

Some older horses may never need drastic modifications to their diet, whereas other senior horses will require a special diet to help them maintain good health and body condition.

The goal is to provide adequate nutrition.

Signs our horses need dental care

Signs a horse may need teeth care include:

- change in eating habits- sometimes refusing to eat or dropping grain out of their mouth
- weight loss
- pain
- drooling
- loose and/or broken teeth
- red, swollen, bleeding, or painful areas in the mouth
- sometimes facial swelling

Seek dental care for any of the above signs and as routine care for a horse's mouth.

The Importance of Dental Care all the Horse's Life

To avoid all the abnormalities of uncared for teeth- wave mouth, slant teeth, abscesses, loss of teeth – resulting in overgrown teeth on the opposing side, shearing of the teeth, and other disorders, regular care is recommended.

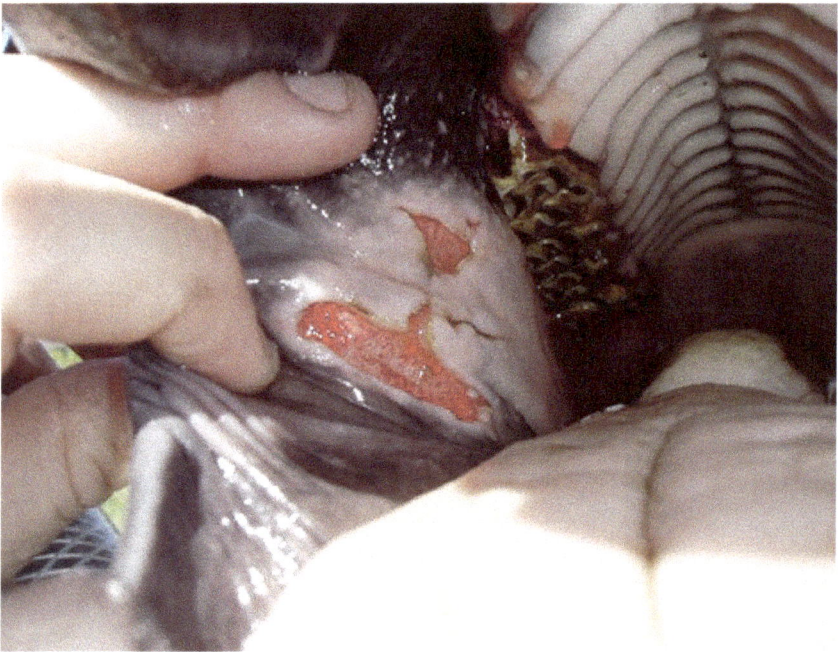

All abnormalities of the mouth and teeth can cause pain, difficulty chewing, loss of nutrition.

Chapter 7

Nutrition

Proper nutrition can:
- help horses live longer
- help prevent dental disease and overweight horses
- help prevent arthritis and the pain associated with arthritis

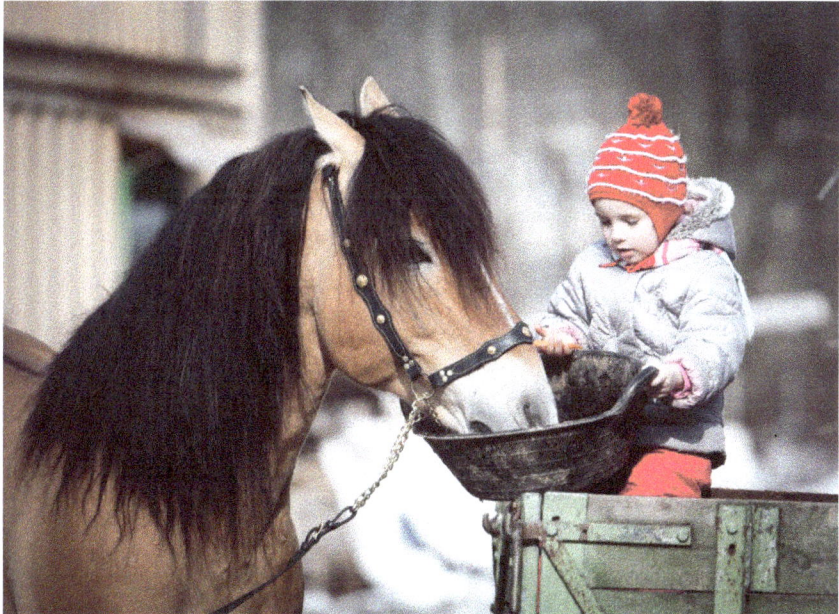

The GOAL in providing nutrition: is to provide proper nutrition for horses for all stages of pet development.

OBJECTIVES OF PROPER NUTRITION FOR THE STAGES OF DEVELOPMENT ARE:

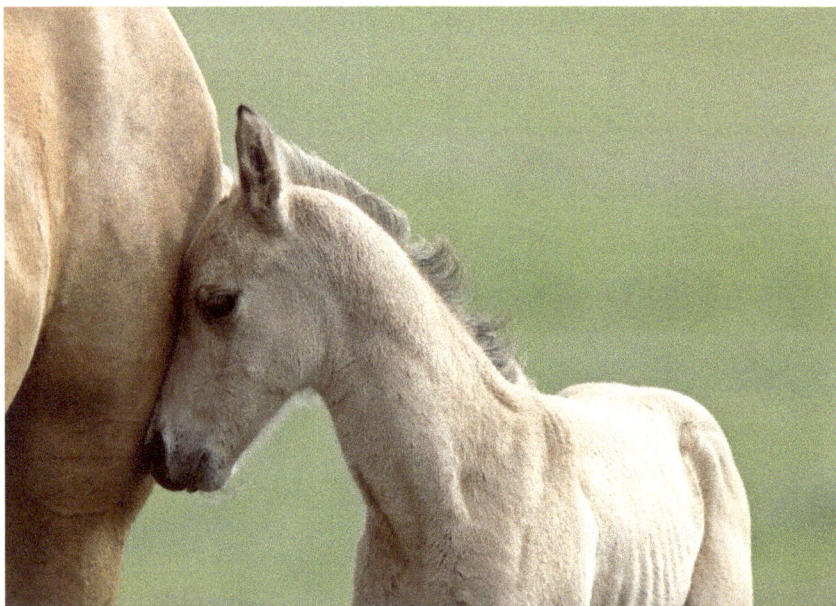

To provide nutrition for body development of young growing foals

- foal supplements are recommended for growing horses

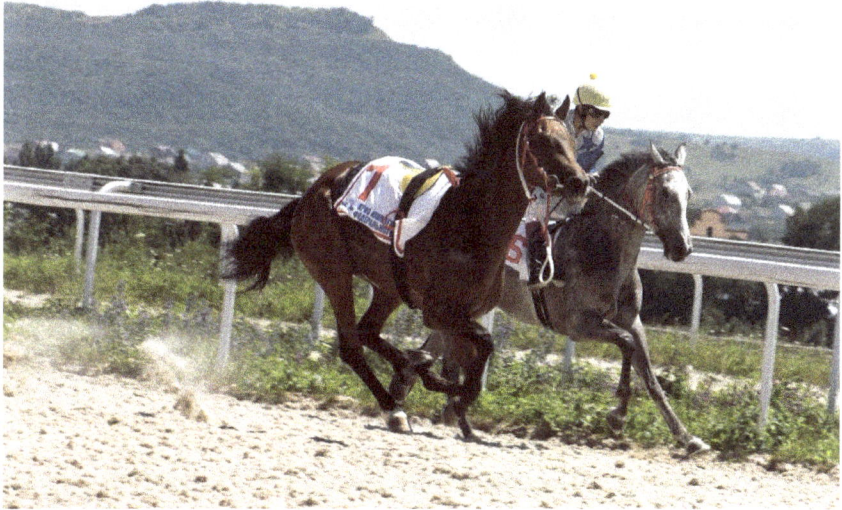

Provide energy for daily activities in young, active, and growing
horses as well as all stages of the horse's life.

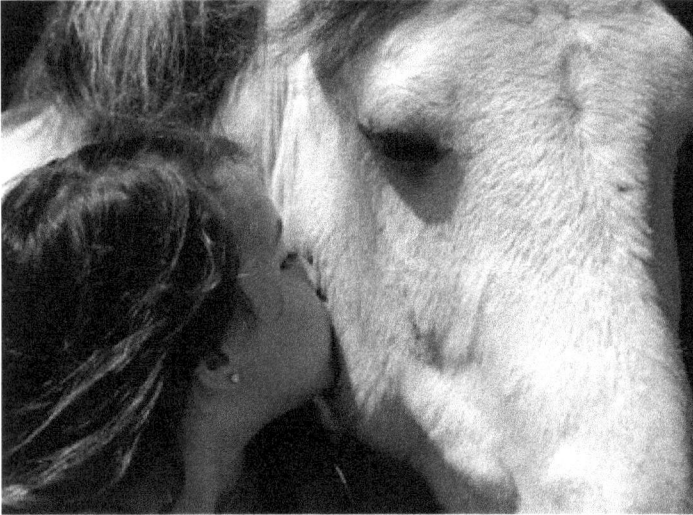

Provide nourishment for a healthy life as they age, including:

- senior diets
- lung care diets
- lameness diets
- overweight management diets
- and more

Horse diets usually consist of:

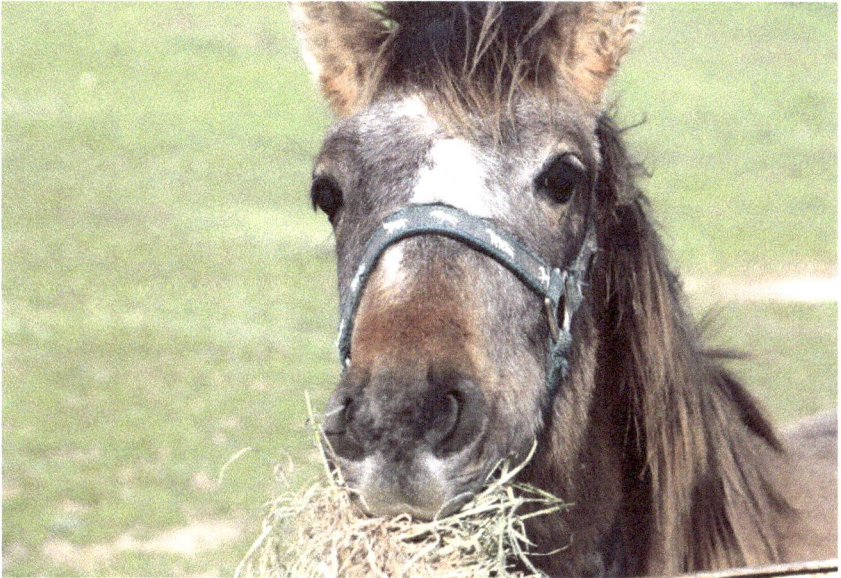

Forages- grass and hay

Concentrates- grain and pelleted rations

Supplements – prepared vitamin and mineral products

Most horse nutritionists recommend at least 50% of the horse's diet be forages. Horses are forage eating animals and are continuous grazing animals in nature- grazing many hours per day.

Horses should have water available always.

THE GOAL of proper nutrition and weight management is -

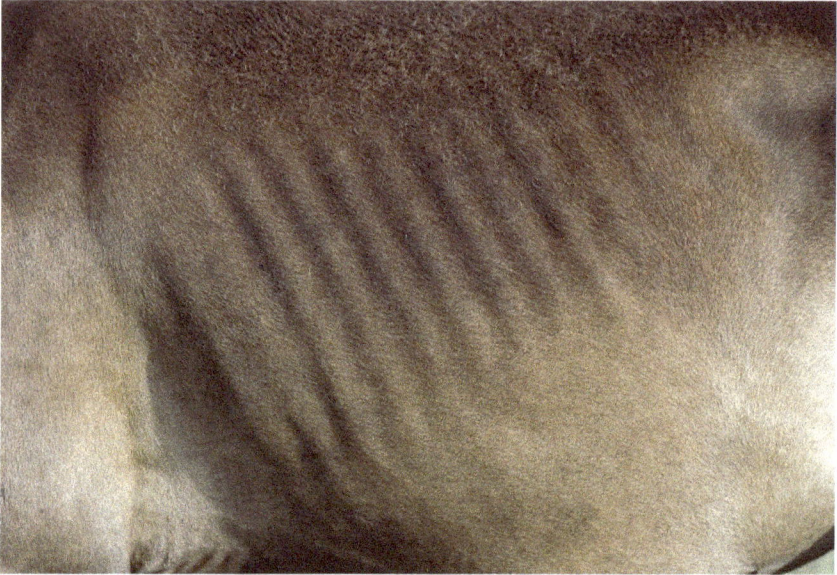

….not too thin…….

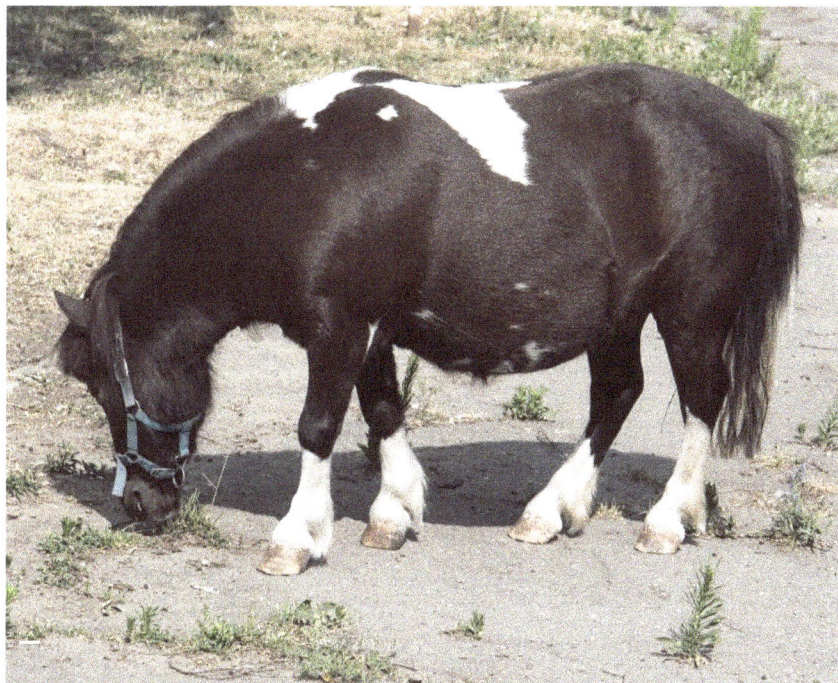

… not too fat …….

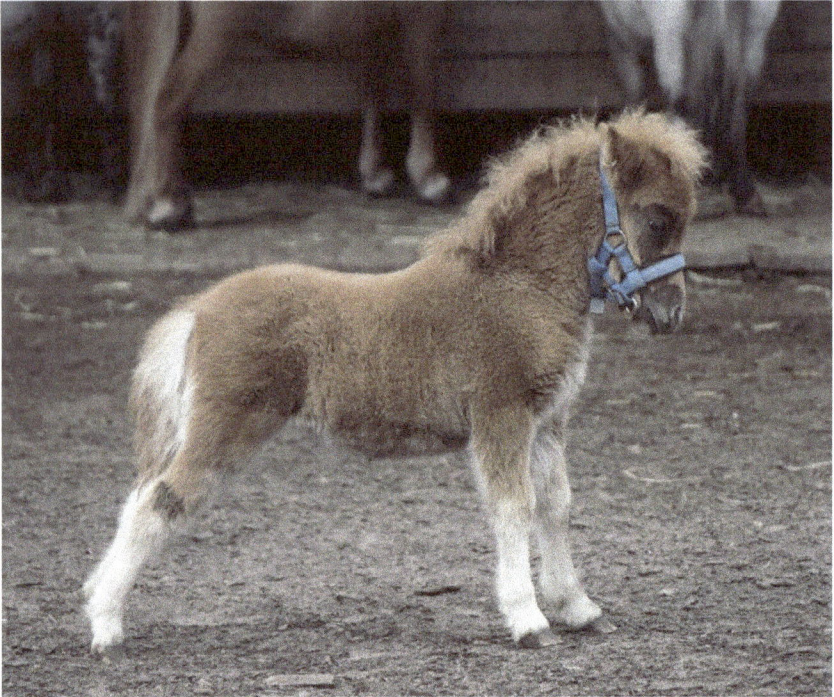

…..but, just right!

Reasons for Healthy Weight in Horses

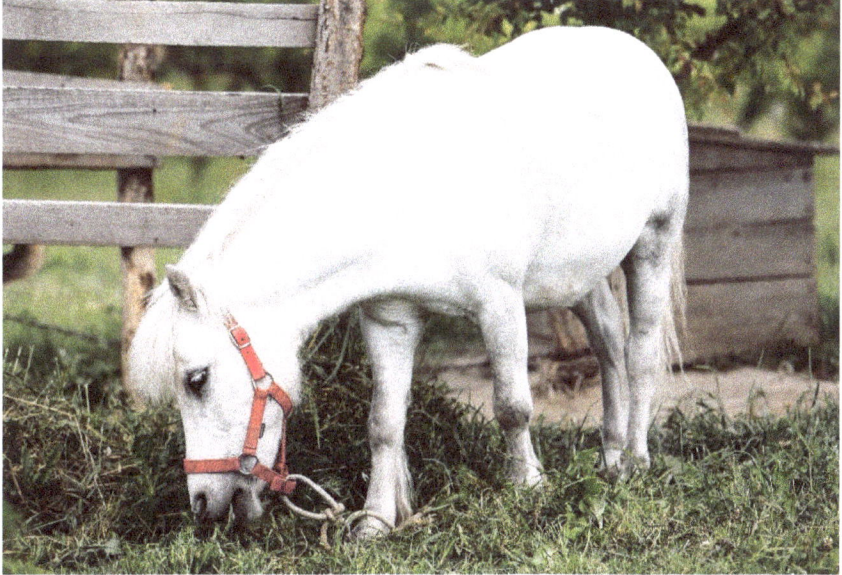

- healthier pets
- easier to exercise
- reduced chance of muscle injuries- tying up syndrome
- increased body weight interferes with cooling in the warm/hot temperatures
- reduced risk of laminitis from excess fat in the abdomen
- overweight horses have more difficulties with reproduction- getting pregnant, maintaining pregnancy, and delivering foals
- overweight horses have higher incidences of heart, blood vessel, digesting, and skin disorders as well as cancer
- overweight horses have shorter life spans

Seek veterinary recommendations for weight loss strategies.

TREATS

Many riders reward their horses with small treats after riding. It makes a profound impact on the horse to be rewarded for 'good' work.

Some guidelines to consider when selecting the type of treat to give the horse include: .

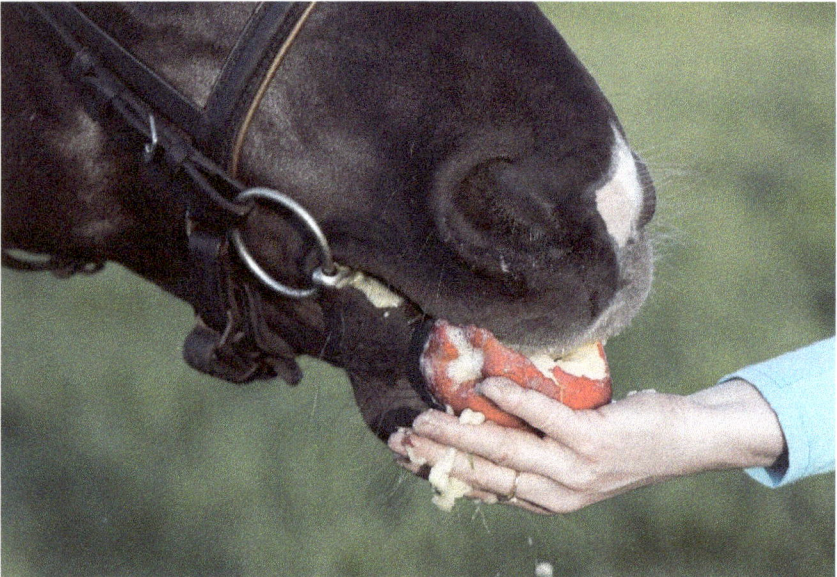

- select healthy vegetables and fruits – these taste good and are close to foods they eat in their normal diet, so will decrease the chance of upsetting their digestive system
- feed small or moderate amounts - too much of certain treats can lead to severe digestive upset and even colic or laminitis

.

What are Good Treats?

- healthy snacks - apple slices, carrots, watermelon, and hay cubes are good choices – some horses will even enjoy a banana

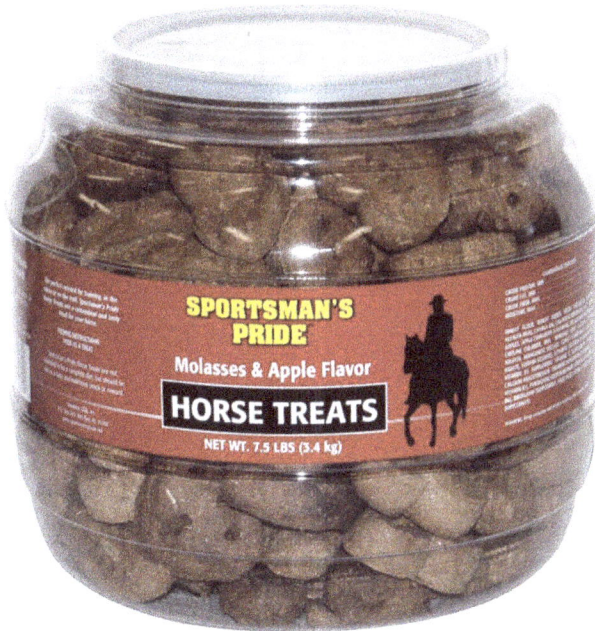

- commercially made horse treats are a favorite for many horses and they may store and travel better than fresh fruit or vegetables when on the road
- sugar cubes and peppermints are traditional treats
- some owners make homemade treats

What Treats Shouldn't Be Fed?

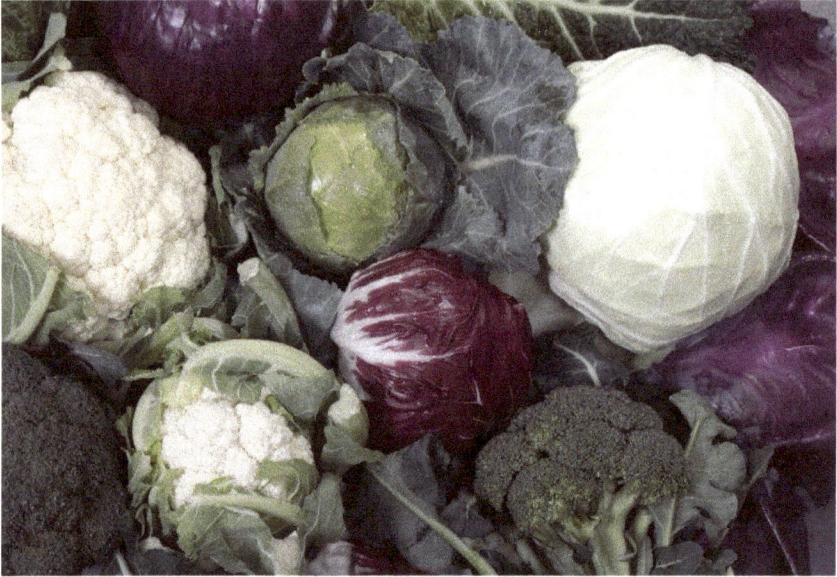

- avoid lawn clippings because these can contain poisonous plants, can cause choke, and can drastically change the acid balance of the intestine – the colon
- avoid cabbage, broccoli, and cauliflower – these can cause severe gas in the intestines if fed in substantial amounts
- avoid potatoes and tomatoes - these are fed by some who feed these with no issues, but it is best to avoid them
- don't feed the pits of fruits because these can cause choke
- chocolate may be enjoyed by a horse, but chocolate can cause a positive result in a drug test
- avoid fresh bread, donuts, and similar foods -these can cause a blockage in the intestines

Chapter 8

Lameness/Arthritis

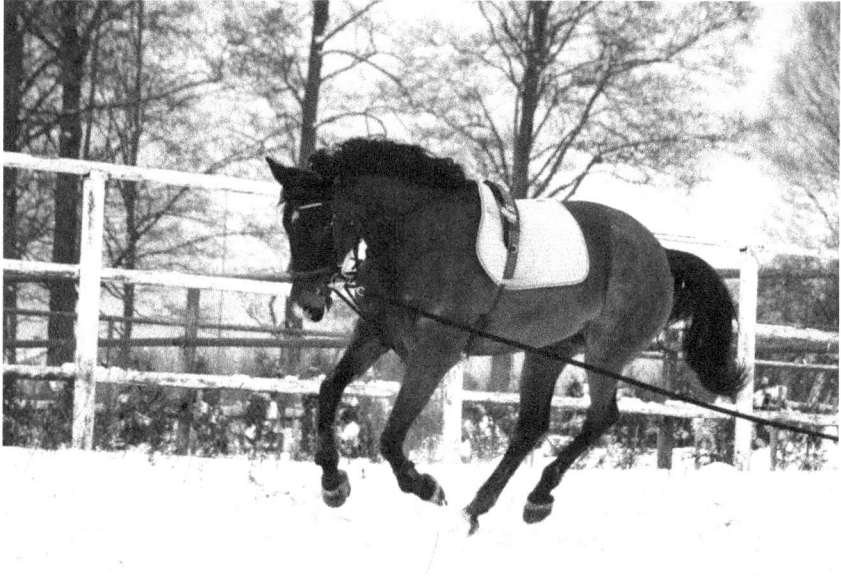

Lameness is a common concern for owners.

Lameness - is any abnormal stance or gait caused by injury or disorders of the muscles and/or bones of the horse.

Lameness is the most common cause of loss of use in horses.

Lameness is not a disease in itself- it is a sign of something causing the lameness - it is a manifestation of pain.

This chapter not only addresses the varied reasons lameness occurs, but is intended to help owners know different disorders and how to identify them when purchasing horses.

135

Causes of lameness include:

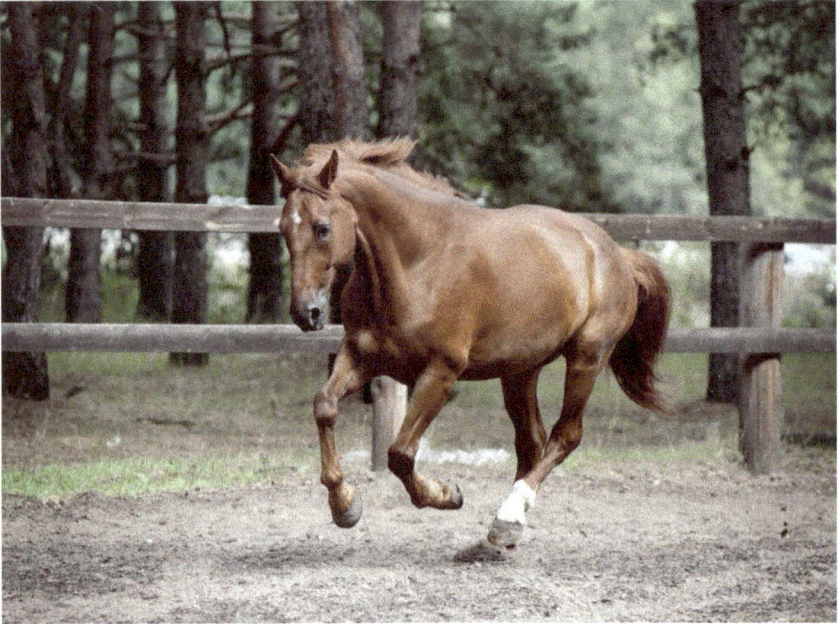

- trauma - injury
- birth abnormalities
- growing disorders of bones and tendons
- infection
- nerve injuries
- blood vessel disease
- and others

Disorders causing lameness include:

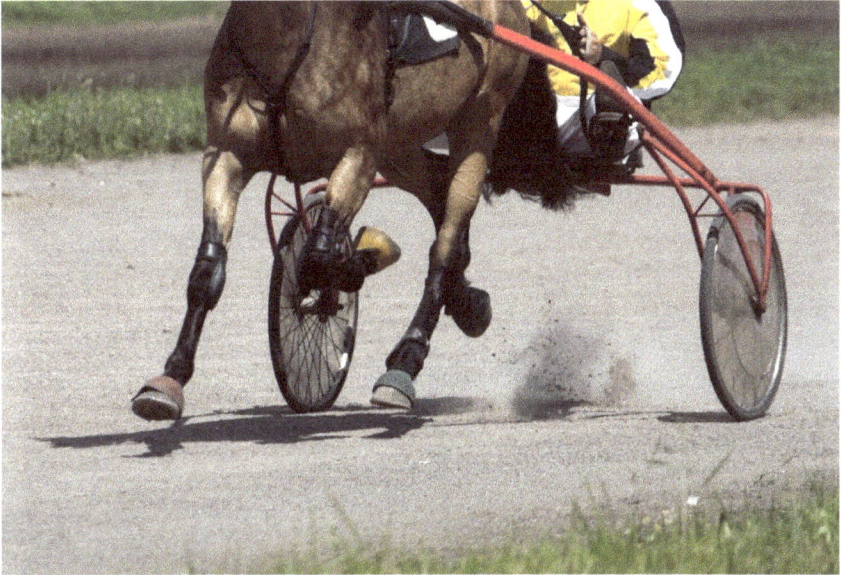

- osteochondrosis (OCD)
- arthritis – ringbone and osselets
- laminitis (founder)
- navicular disease
- bowed tendons
- strains/sprains
- thrush
- punctures of the foot
- cuts – including cuts of tendons
- broken bones
- muscle tension – from overwork to ill-fitting equipment
- sore feet –for many reasons-including bare feet on rough surfaces
- ill-fitting shoes
- and more

Signs of lameness include-

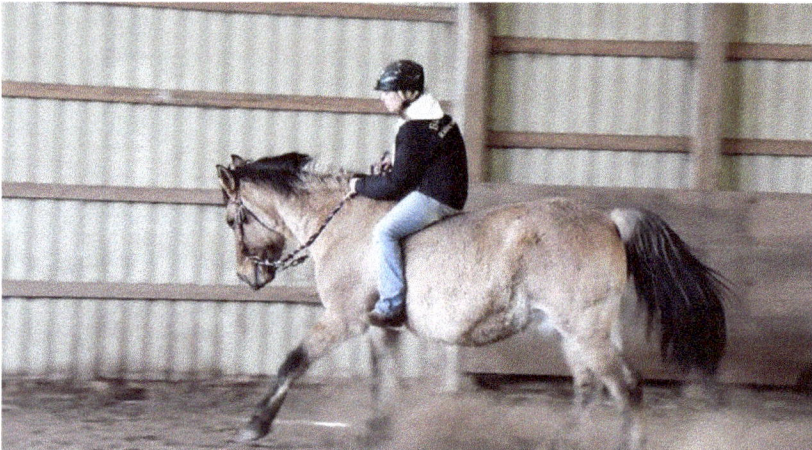

- unwillingness to stand or move normally
- limping
- deformity in the leg/legs – as in broken bones or growth abnormalities
- swelling
- pain when touched
- discharge that is white/green/yellow/or tan- with an odor
- open sores

Completing a lameness exam includes:

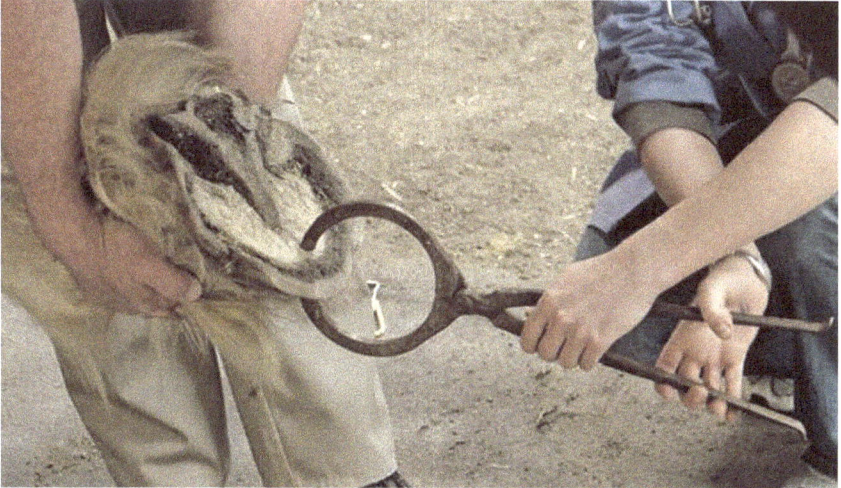

- watching the horse move – whether on a lead rope, a lounge line, or under saddle
- watching the horse walk, trot, and canter after bending joints- flexing and extending the various joints of the front and back legs
- touching the various parts of the body- especially the muscles of the neck and back and upper legs- evaluating these areas for any pain
- having a veterinarian block nerves with medication and then observing the horsewalking, trotting, and cantering
- x-rays or ultrasound - many views may be necessary for the x-rays to find bone disorders

DO NOT exercise a horse if a broken bone is suspected – this could lead to catastrophe.

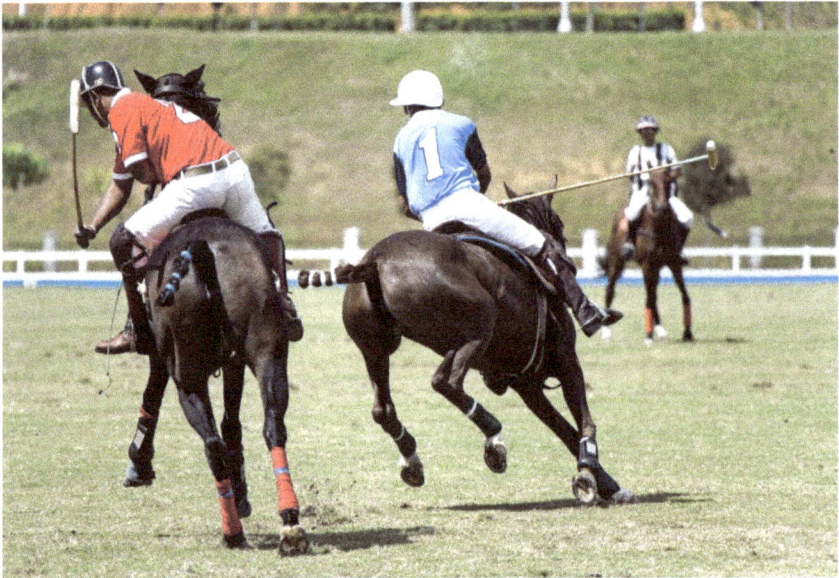

Also remember, it is impossible to evaluate a heavily sedated horse, however, sometime mild sedation is necessary.

Osteochondrosis-(OCD)

Osteochondrosis-(OCD) (oss – tee- oh – kon- drow- sis) - is a disorder involving bones and cartilage in young growing horses.

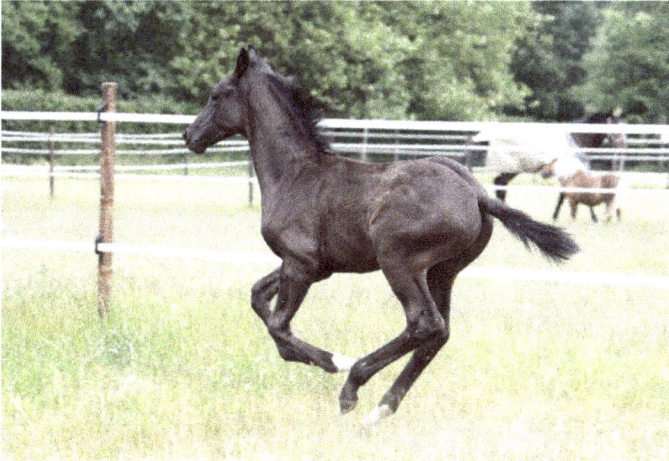

In normal bone formation, bone begins as cartilage and changes to bone as the bones grow and develop. In OCD, the cartilage does not change to bone properly and since cartilage does not have a direct blood supply, the extra cartilage is not healthy and results in cartilage 'flaps' or sloughs from the ends of the bones.

This cartilage can break loose and float in the joint space- between the affected bones. This causes arthritis – which results in pain and lameness if not corrected surgically.

It is not certain exactly why this disorder occurs, however,

- rapid growth
- excess carbohydrates in the diet
- genetics
- and trauma due to overexertion

....are some of the speculated causes.

Another cause is mineral imbalance.

Signs of ostesochondrosis include

- swelling of a joint (where two bones come together) - in many horse the swelling is not painful

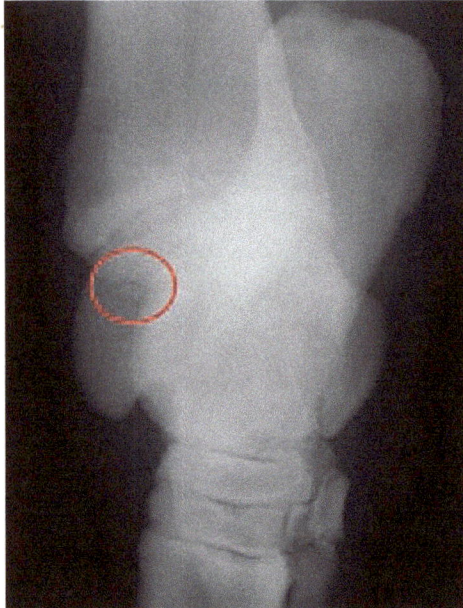

- x-ray evidence of cartilage fragments in the joint – as above
- lameness if allowed to progress

Prevention includes proper nutrition for pregnant and nursing mares as well as nutritional supplementation for the foal.

Seek the advice of a veterinarian if you have young growing horses.

Additional Disorders in Young Growing Horses

Other disorders that may occur in young growing horses include:

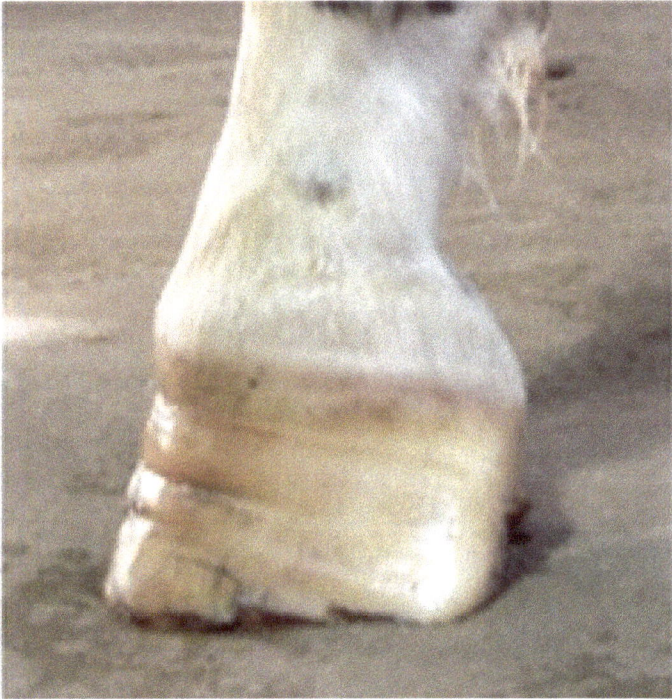

- angular limb deformity
- cervical (neck) vertebral instability (wobbler)
- contracted tendons
- club foot- noted above
- and more

Disorders of the foot are numerous, including –

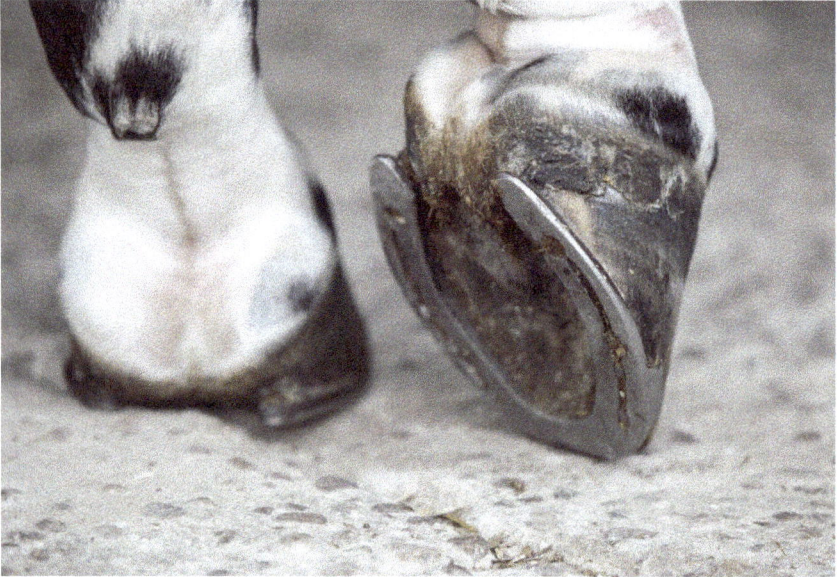

- laminitis
- navicular disease
- puncture wounds
- bruises
- infections (abscess)
- thrush
- fractured (broken) bones
- and others

The horse's foot and ankle are made of several bones and joints.

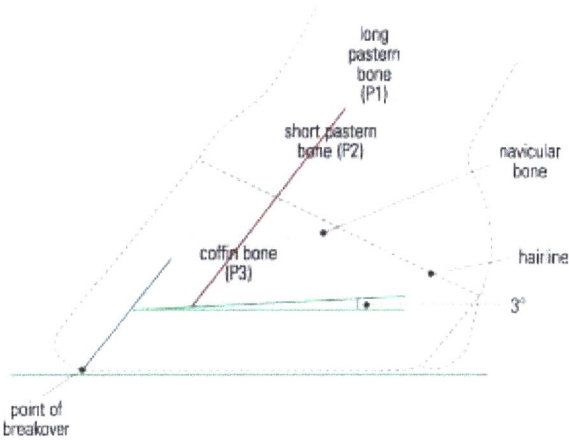

long
pastern
bone
(P1)

short pastern
bone (P2)

navicular
bone

coffin bone
(P3)

hair ine

3°

point of
breakover

Normal structures of the lower leg and foot.

LAMINITIS (FOUNDER)

Laminitis in horses – (lam- in- eye- tis) also known as founder - is a crippling disease in which there is a breakdown in the attachment of the hoof wall to the underlying bone in the feet.

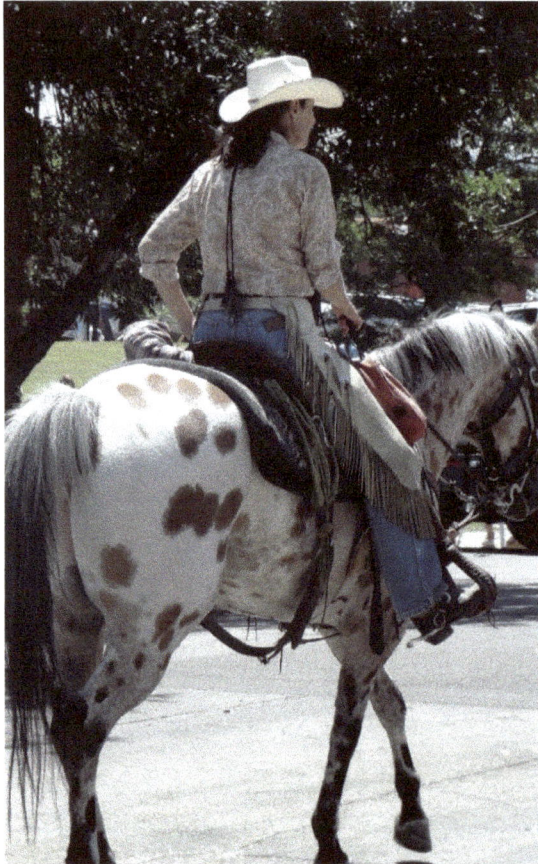

The hoof wall attaches to the 'coffin' bone and keeps it in the foot in the proper place. If this attachment is altered, the bone shifts and there is great danger of the bone displacing downward and coming out of the bottom of the sole of the hoof. If this extreme loss of connection between this last bone and the hoof wall happens, the horse will be lost.

Laminitis may affect all breeds of horses.

146

Several causes of laminitis are thought to be:

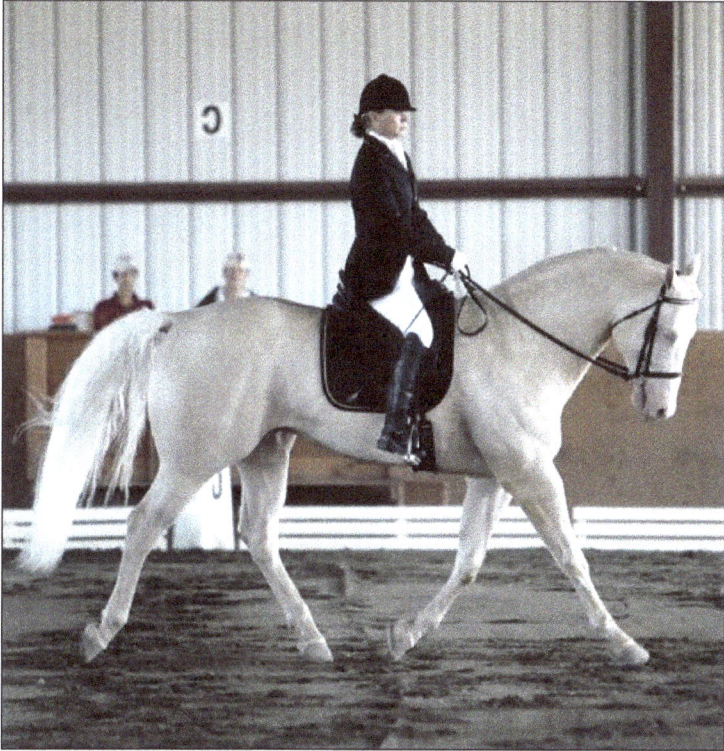

- diseases with infection that spreads throughout the body - known as sepsis or endotoxemia – bacterial infection is the most common
- overeating grain -laminitis occurs because of the high sugars in the feed
- retained placentas in mares after foal delivery
- or metritis (infection of the uterus) after foal delivery
- colic for any reason
- intestinal twisting

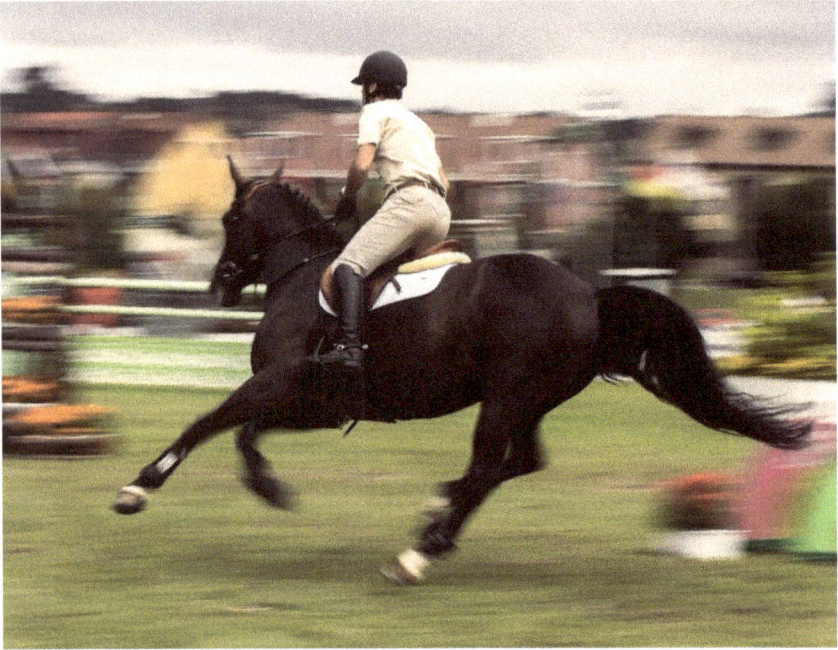

(more causes of laminitis)

- overweight conditions in horses
- grazing in lush pastures – especially new grass in the spring without slowly adjusting to the pasture grass
- high or low temperature events – such as over exposure to the cold or heat
- hormonal disorders which includes equine metabolic syndrome (including pasture-associated laminitis) and pituitary gland (a small gland in the brain) masses
- supporting limb laminitis- when a horse places more weight on a leg due to pain on an alternative leg, this pressure causes injury to the hoof wall
- ingestion of or exposure to shavings used for bedding (not intended for bedding) such as black walnut heartwood

There are three manifestations of laminitis:

Acute - which is a sudden, new occurrence of laminitis – usually the first few days - < 3 days.

In the acute phase, there is no displacement of bone in the hoof- the third phalangeal bone - the coffin bone.

Subacute – which is when the signs of laminitis last longer than 3 days.

In the subacute phase, there is still no displacement of the bone in the hoof- the third phalangeal bone- the coffin bone.

Chronic- which is when displacement of the coffin bone has occurred to one degree or another.

Signs of laminitis include:

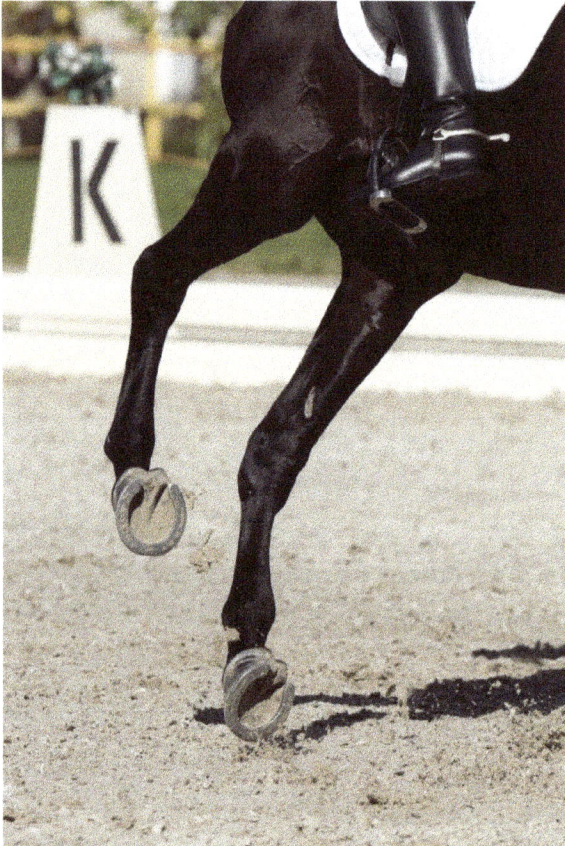

- lameness – pain – which may be slight limping to being unable to walk – some horses with laminitis stand with their feet stretched forward if only the front feet are affected to decrease the pain of pressure on the feet
- increased pulses to the foot may be noted by feeling the pulse on the sides of the ankles
- additional signs of pain are an increase heart rate (60-120) and breathing rate (80-100)
- warmth to the hoof walls may be noted
- sometimes horses show a crouched appearance
- some horses take short steps if all 4 feet are affected

(additional signs of laminitis)

- tenderness to the hoof wall when pressed with a hoof tester – a tool veterinarians and blacksmiths use

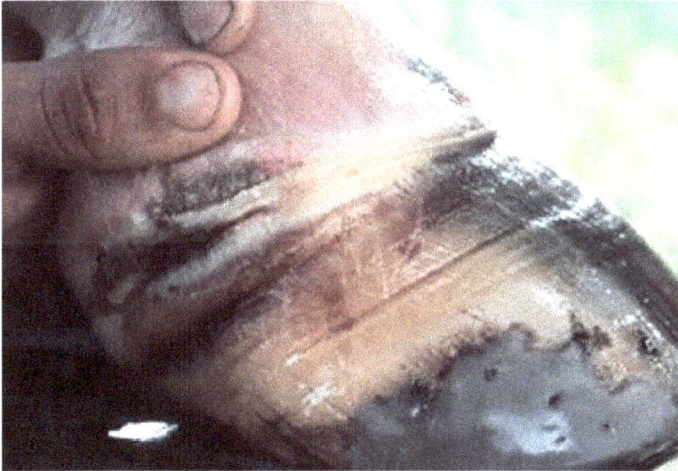

- the horse may be down and not able to get up
- over long time- changes in the hoof wall may be noted- such as irregular ridges appear on the hoof wall

Diagnosing laminitis –

In acute laminitis - diagnosis is usually straightforward and is based on the history (e.g., grain overload) and posture of the horse, increased temperature of the hooves, a strong pulse in the digital arteries, and reluctance to move.

Acute laminitis constitutes a medical emergency, because phalangeal bone displacement can occur rapidly. One must understand that the outcome is not predictable until recovery is complete and it is evident that the hoof structure is not altered.

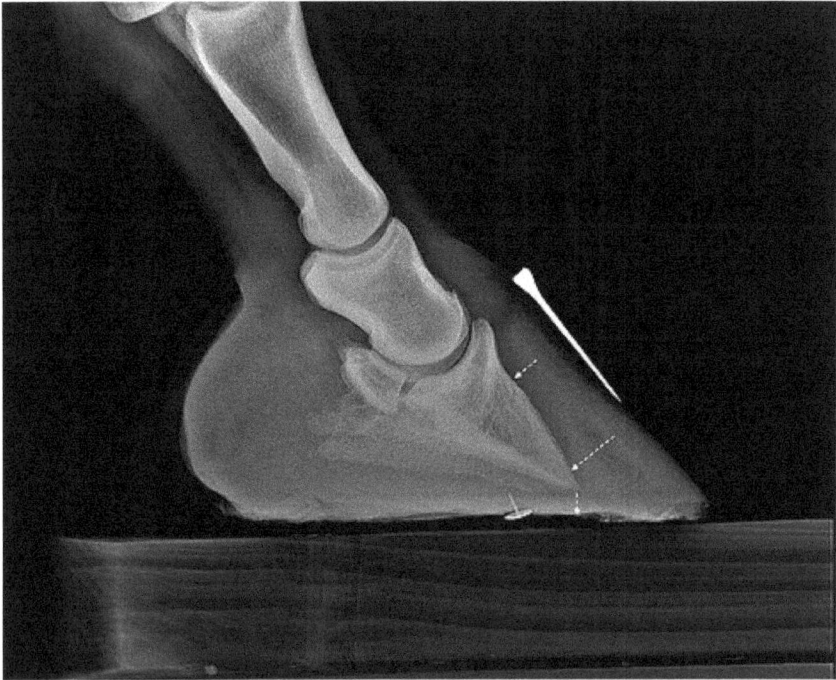

X-rays determine movement of the bones inside the horse's foot.

Seek veterinary care for horses with the signs of laminitis.

NAVICULAR

Navicular disease is a chronic (longstanding) degenerative condition in the navicular bone …

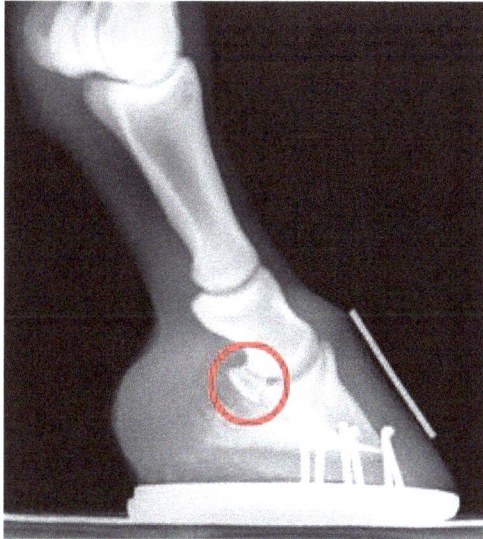

……. which lies behind and under the small pastern bone. The navicular bone acts as a fulcrum that the tendon that attaches to the coffin bone runs over.

Navicular is the most common cause of lameness in the front leg of athletic horses, but is not usually seen in ponies or donkeys.

Causes and contributing factors - there is no single known cause of navicular syndrome, but there are many thoughts on what causes it as well as several common factors – some include:

:

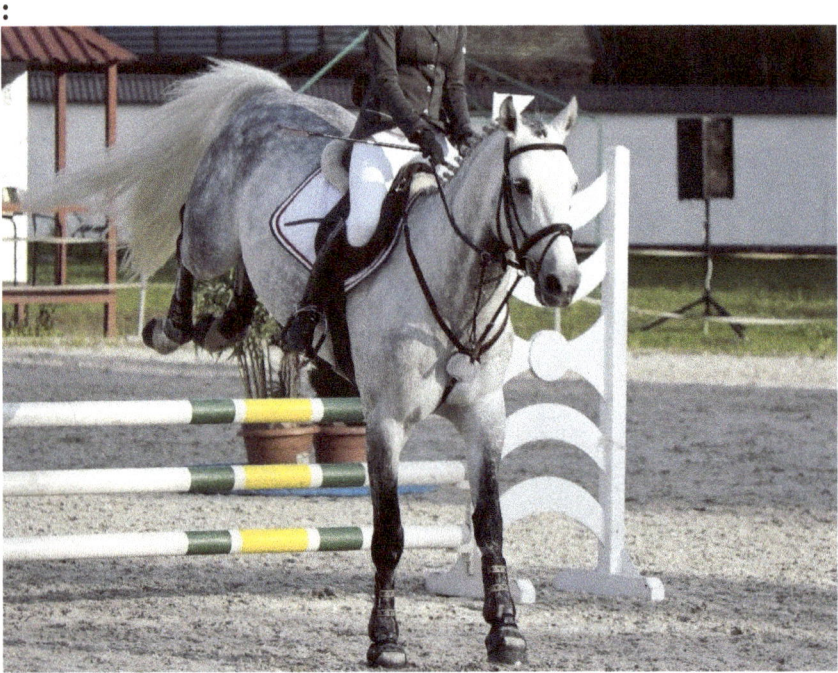

- compression of the navicular bone against the back of the small pastern bone under the tendon that attaches to the coffin bone
- repeated compression in this area can cause cartilage degeneration, with the cartilage flattening and gradually becoming less springy and shock-absorbing – the cartilage may also begin to erode
- cartilage degeneration is common in navicular horses and this, along with the chemical changes in the bone, have led some to conclude that navicular disease is like a form of arthritis

(additional contributing factors for navicular)

- the cartilage may erode to the point that the bone underneath becomes exposed – this can damage the tendon that rides over this bone and worsen the pain
- navicular bursitis (inflammation of the navicular bursa- the delicate lining over the navicular bone) may occur, even if cartilage damage is not severe- this may be due to the friction between the navicular bone and the tendon compressing over the bone
- constant compression by the tendon may increase the thickness of the bone under the cartilage surfaces which may make the bone more brittle and more easily broken
- another main factor is the tension placed on the ligaments that support the navicular bone, causing strain and irritation – and irritation from strain of the impar ligament can decrease blood flow to and from the navicular bone
- excess tension may cause extra bone growth that appears as jagged edges of bone instead of smooth surfaces- when this occurs, the ligaments attaching to the navicular bone may tear
- improper shoeing may contribute to navicular and veterinarians and blacksmiths need to be consulted for recommendations for proper shoeing so the horse lands properly on the foot while exercising
- certain conformational defects may contribute to navicular syndrome - especially defects that promote concussion (hitting the foot hard and improperly) such as upright pasterns, small feet, narrow and upright feet, significant downhill build seen in some breeds of horses
- working on steep hills, galloping, and jumping all contribute to navicular syndrome, as they place greater stress on the tendons over the navicular bone and cause overextension of the pastern and coffin joints

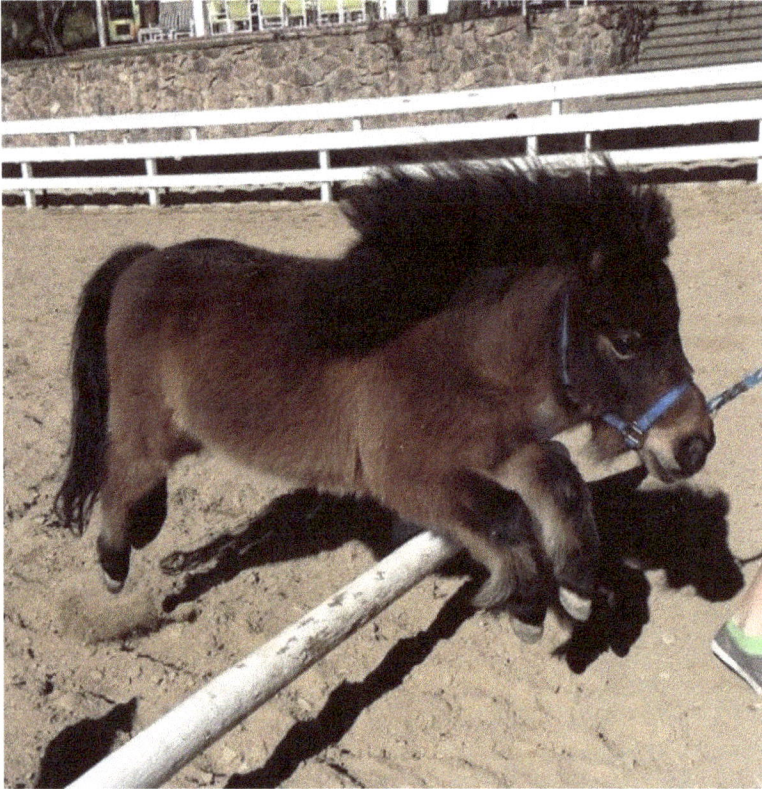

- regular exercise on hard or irregular ground increases concussion on the hoof – increasing the risk of navicular syndrome
- it is possible that standing can also increase the chance of navicular disease (such as a horse that spends most of the day in a stall with little turnout) because blood flow decreases to the hoof when the horse is not in motion and pressure is constant to the navicular bones (which pressure is typically intermittent as the horse moves)
- horses with a high weight-to-foot-size ratio may have an increased chance of navicular syndrome because there is greater load on the foot

Signs of Navicular Include:

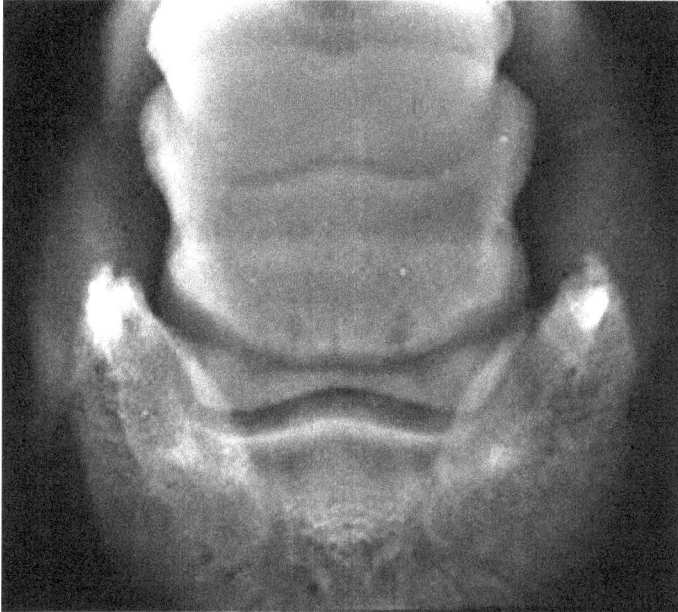

- heel pain is common in horses with navicular
- lameness may begin as mild and occasional and progress to severe and constant – and may be worse when worked on a firm surface or in a circle
- affected horses have a "tiptoe" gait - trying to walk on the toes due to heel pain and may stumble frequently
- lameness may switch from one leg to another and may not be consistent - lameness usually occurs in both front feet, although one foot may be more affected than the other
- after several months of pain, the feet may begin to change shape - becoming more upright and narrow
- affected horses are pain free -not lame - with nerve blocks
- usually both front feet are affected
- x-rays may show many different amounts of bone changes involving the navicular bone

Treatment and long term outcome

It is important to note that navicular is a degenerative disease and cannot be cured, but can be managed.

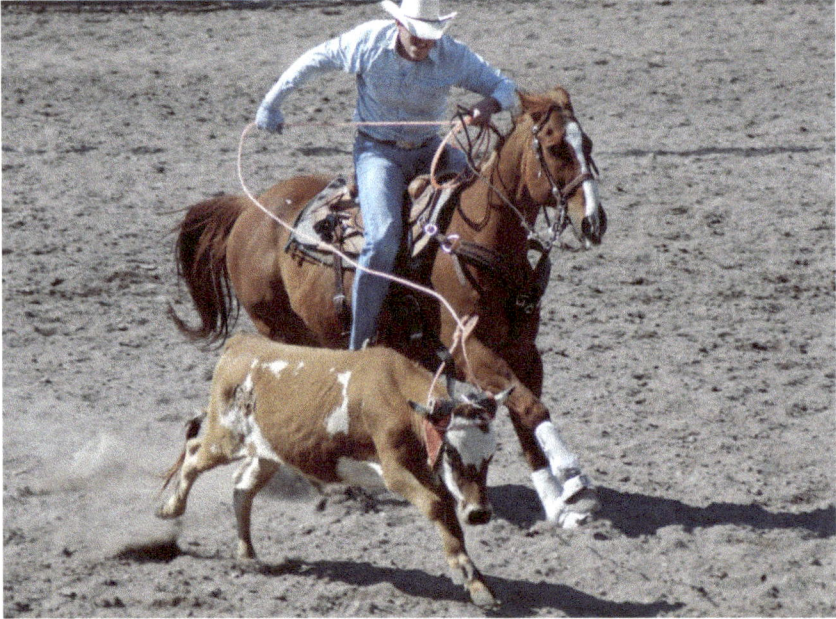

Seek veterinary and farrier care for a horse with navicular disease for exercise, shoeing, and care recommendations.

PUNCTURE WOUNDS and ABSCESSES

Puncture wounds – occur when any object penetrates the foot or skin of the horse.

Puncture wounds are common in horses and are the most common cause of foot infection (abscess).

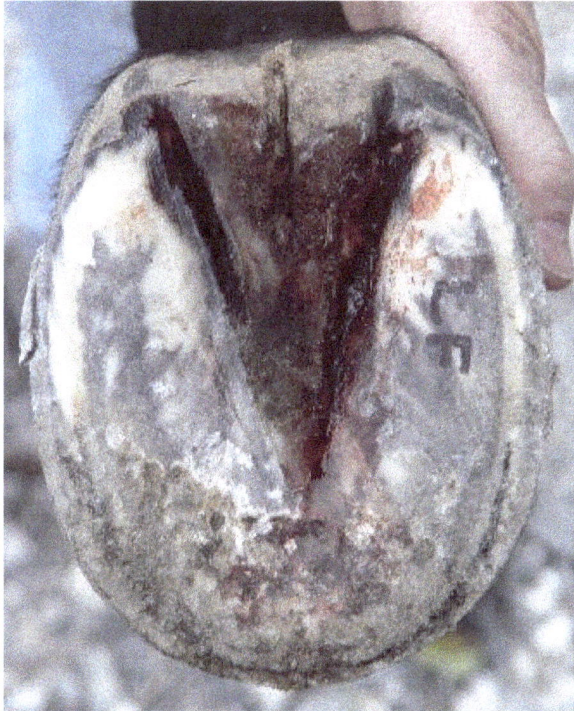

Most puncture wounds only result in infection (abscess) of the subsolar soft tissue (the area under the sole of the foot).

Foot abscesses are easily drained by a veterinarian or blacksmith by cutting into the affected sole and allowing drainage. Soaking and/or poultice may be used for after care

Even though most abscesses are easily treated, if the puncture is in the frog and travels deep enough to enter the bones or the linings around the bones or tendons in the foot, this is catastrophic.

Signs of puncture wounds/foot abscesses include:

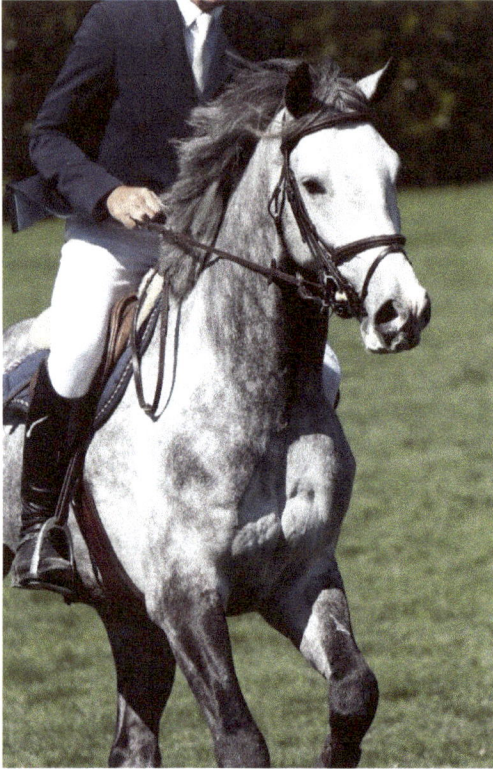

- lameness that is usually severe – as severe as that of a broken bone
- the horse may stand pointing the affected foot
- there is commonly a prominent digital pulse in the affected limb
- if allowed to progress, the abscess may travel up the hoof wall and rupture at the coronary band (known as a gravel)
- and there will usually be swelling at the coronary band (the hair line) before rupture of the gravel
- if the infection is deep, then the deep structures of the foot and ankle may be swollen, warm, and painful to the touch as well as the lameness will be severe

Diagnosis of foot abscess-

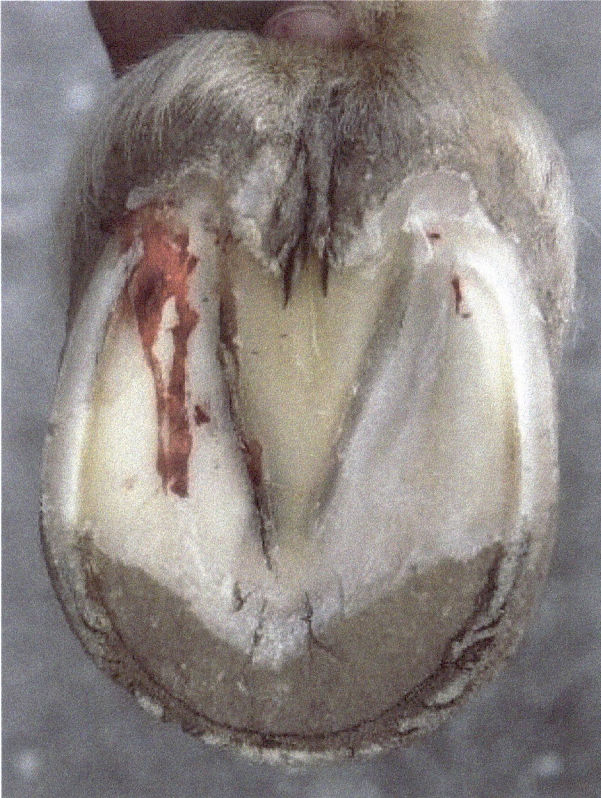

- is made by confirming the site of pain by pulling the shoe, using hoof testers, and picking or paring the suspect area to locate the foreign body or its dark tract
- if a foreign body is found in the frog, it may be best to obtain an x-ray of the foot to assess the structures penetrated before removing the offending object
- if a tract of infection is found in the frog, it should be probed and an x-ray taken with the probe in place to evaluate deeper structures

Penetrating objects to the frog are serious because puncture wounds in or near the frog commonly enter a lining around a bone in the foot and require rapid, aggressive diagnosis and therapy.

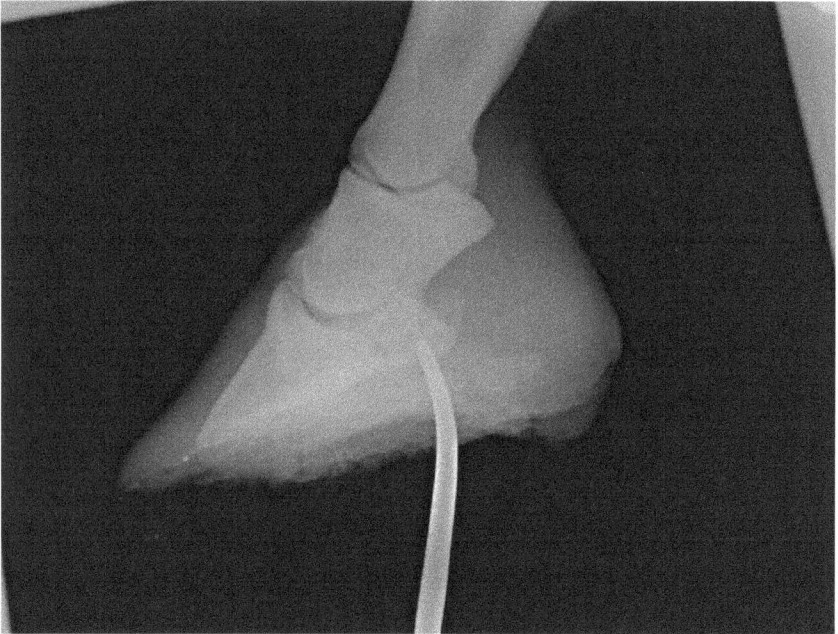

Penetrating foot injuries may lead to loss of a horse.

Ask your veterinarian for all after care for foot abscesses and make certain the horse has tetanus protection.

THRUSH

Thrush - is a degeneration of the frog with bacterial and fungal infection. The affected parts become moist and have a black, thick discharge with a characteristic foul odor. Parts of the frog may be necrotic (dead tissue).

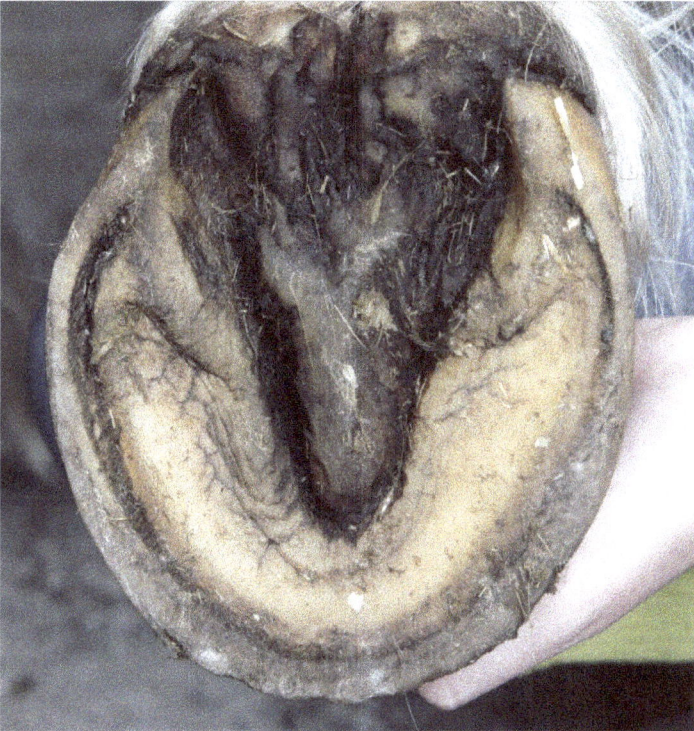

Many consider the cause of thrush to be a moist environment with poor hygiene, however, other factors may contribute to thrush.

No matter the cause, a moist environment should be avoided in animals with thrush.

The signs of thrush are sufficient to make the diagnosis.

Ask your veterinarian for treatment recommendations and provide a dry, clean flooring and thorough cleaning of the frog and sulci.

OSSELETS

Osselets--it's an outdated term for a disorder involving the ankles (fetlock joints) of the horse. It begins as a thickening of the joint tissues in the front of the fetlock joints – usually in the front legs.

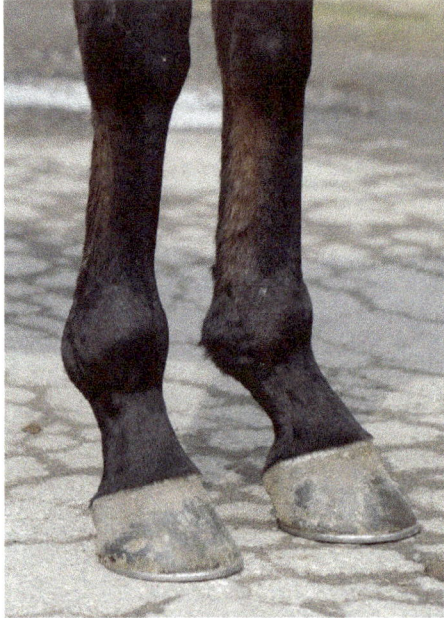

Osselets may progress to arthritis and sometimes have calcium deposits in the tissue in front of the fetlocks which cause irritation to the joint which causes pain in the horse.

Osselets are caused by trauma - such as when racing horses or jumping horses land heavily on their front legs.

Other working horses can experience overuse of the front legs- such as barrel horses, cutting horses, 3-day event horses, and others.

Signs of Osselets include:

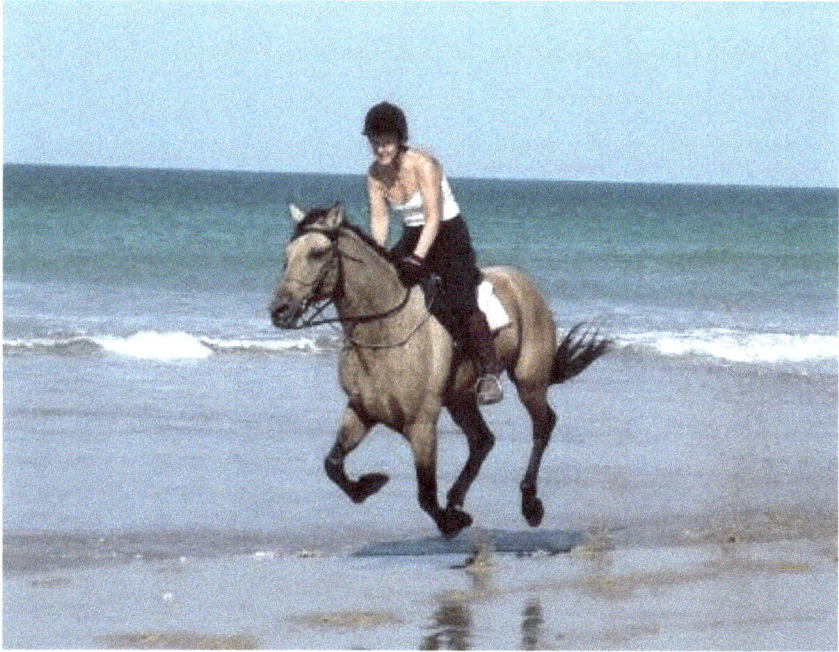

- swelling and warmth to the front of the front fetlocks in the early phases (known as green osselets)
- sometimes swelling develops to the sides of the fetlock joint as well (known commonly as windpuffs)
- with time, lameness may develop- especially when the fetlock joint is flexed and the horse is watched walking or trotting afterwards
- when lame, the gait is usually short and chopping
- if the horse continues to work, arthritis is possible - once arthritis develops, there is no cure and life- long management is necessary with pain medication and rest

Diagnosis of osselets includes:

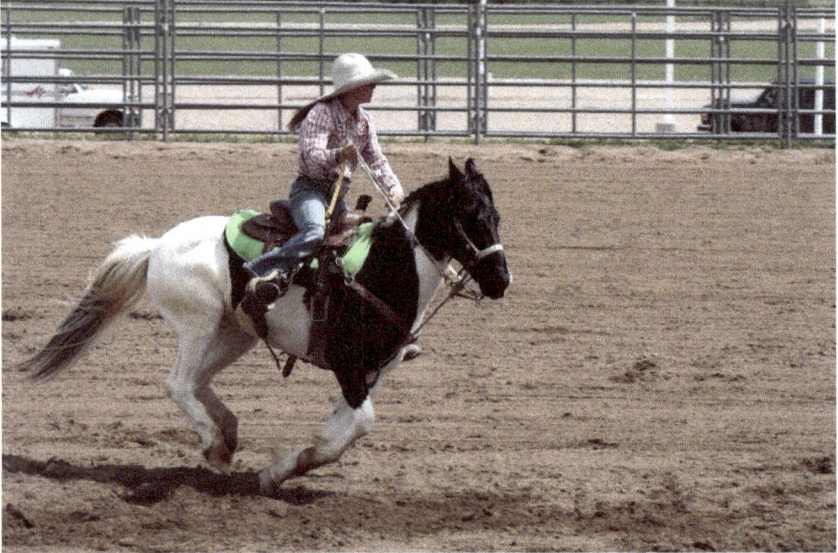

- a lameness exam – that demonstrates pain on flexion
- or pain when one presses on the affected front aspects of the fetlock (ankle)
- a short choppy gait when both front fetlocks are involved
- lack of lameness with the use of nerve blocks completed by a veterinarian
- x-rays may help determine if injury to the bone has occurred

It is important to diagnose osselets early because, as with many arthritic conditions, the sooner osselets are detected, the more successful treatment is.

RINGBONE

Ringbone- is a horseman's term for arthritis in the ankle and foot joints.

"High ringbone" is arthritis in the first interphalangeal joint

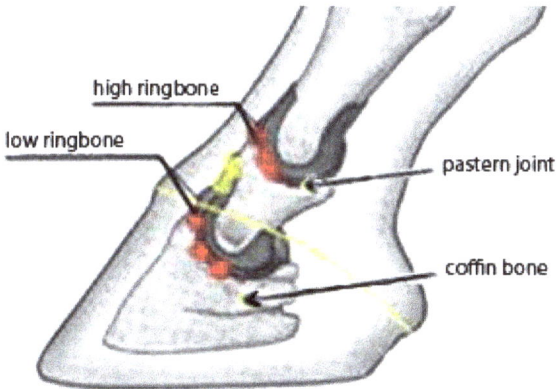

"Low ringbone" is arthritis in the second interphalangeal joint

Arthritis in horses' ankle joints may be from a severe injury that may even cause a 'chip' (small) fracture of the bones of the joint or may be a result of "wear and tear," or overuse.

Other causes of arthritis of these joints are infection and developmental bone disorders – such as osteochondrosis.

Diagnosis of Ringbone:

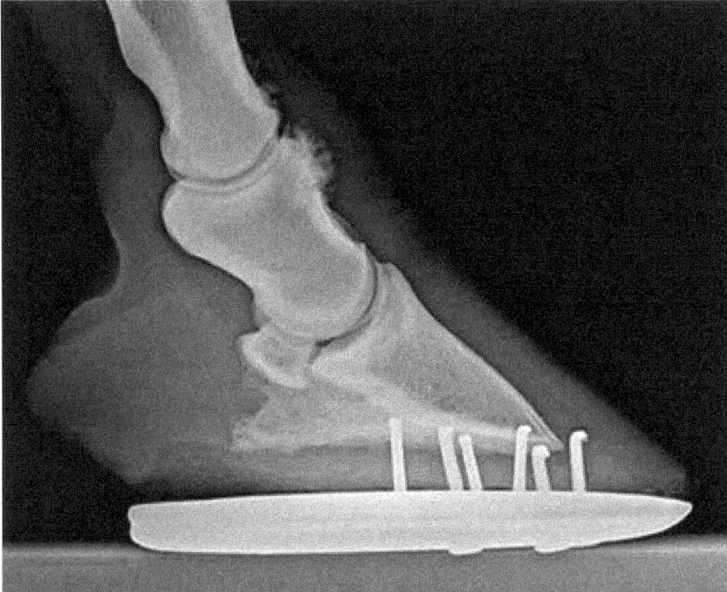

The diagnosis is made by x-ray findings

The horse is usually lame on a lameness exam – especially on flexion of the ankle.

In the initial stages of disease (before it may be detected on x-rays), your veterinarian may complete a nerve block to localize the lameness.

Ask your veterinarian for treatment recommendations.

STRINGHALT

Stringhalt - is a gait abnormality characterized by exaggerated upward flexion of the hindlimb occuring at every stride at the walk.

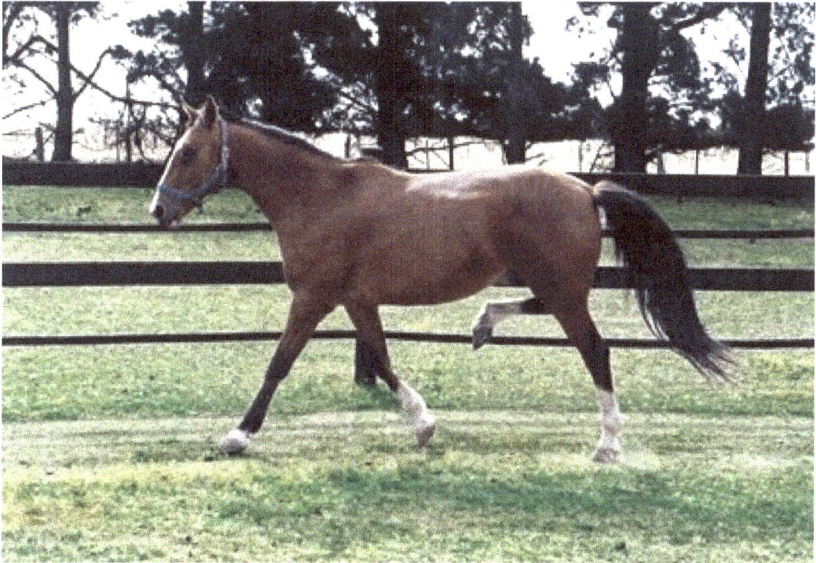

The gait abnormality – stringhalt - usually lessens at the trot and is not evident at canter.

It may occur on only one side of the back legs or both back legs.

All degrees of hyperflexion may be seen - from mild, spasmodic lifting and grounding of the foot, to extreme cases in which the foot is drawn sharply up until it touches the belly and is then struck violently on the ground.

The cause of stringhalt is not known.

Signs of Stringhalt include:

- signs that may be most obvious when the horse is sharply turned or backed
- in some cases, the condition is seen only on the first few steps when moving the horse
- the signs are often less intense or even absent during warmer weather
- in severe cases, there is a decrease in the muscles of the side of the thigh

Although it is regarded as unsoundness, stringhalt may not hinder the horse's ability to work, except in severe cases when the constant concussion gives rise to additional complications like arthritis, laminitis, broken bones, navicular or other disorders.

The condition may make the horse unsuitable for some equestrian disciplines (e.g., dressage).

Diagnosis of stringhalt:

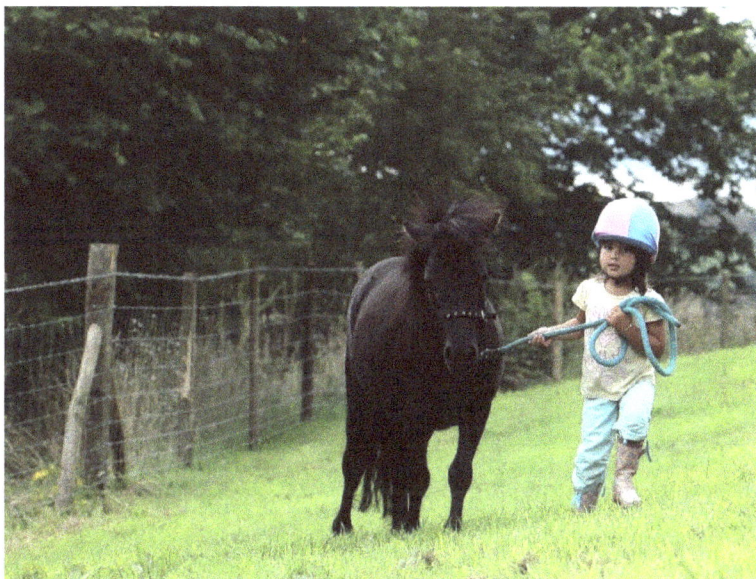

- is based on the signs above, but can be confirmed by electromyography – electrical studies of the muscles
- if the diagnosis is in doubt, the horse should be observed as it is backed out of the stall after vigorous work for 1–2 days
- false stringhalt sometimes appears because of some temporary irritation to the lower pastern area or even a painful lesion in the foot

INJURY TO THE SUSPENSORY LIGAMENTS

Suspensory ligaments are strong fibrous structures that lie behind the 'cannon' bones and are supportive structures to prevent over extension of the fetlock joint during work.

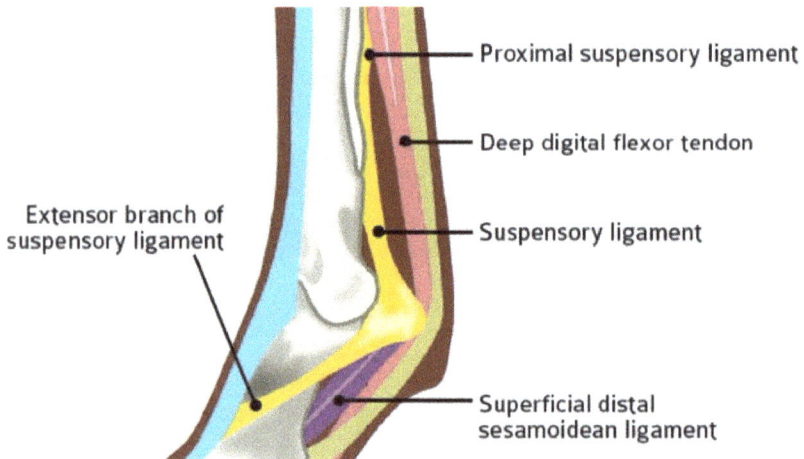

Labels on diagram:
- Proximal suspensory ligament
- Deep digital flexor tendon
- Suspensory ligament
- Superficial distal sesamoidean ligament
- Extensor branch of suspensory ligament

Every horse can injure this supportive structure, however, horses that place great strain on the leg or legs are most at risk – such as racing horses, eventers, and barrel horses.

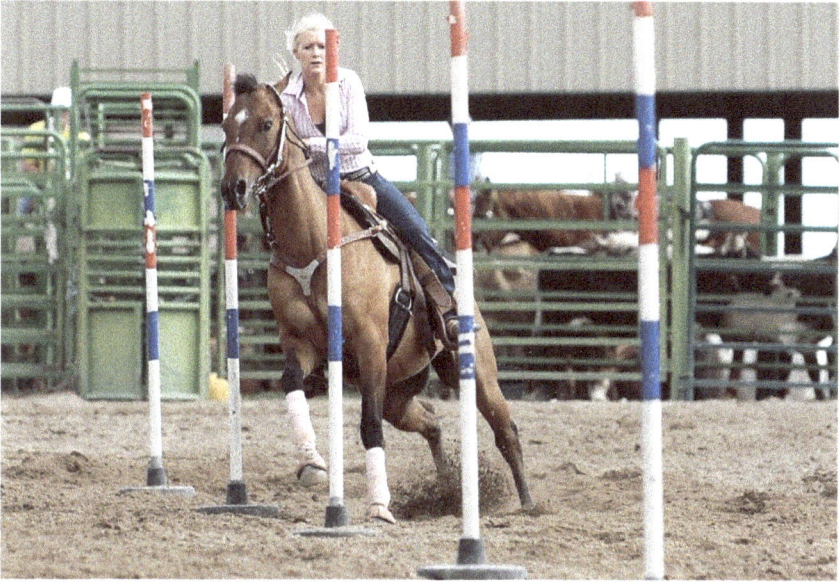

When injured, there may be strain or tearing of the fibers of the suspensory ligament.

Signs include:

- pain
- swelling
- warmth
- lameness – of varying degrees
- and injury to the suspensory ligament may end an athletic career

Diagnosis of suspensory ligaments and tendons ....

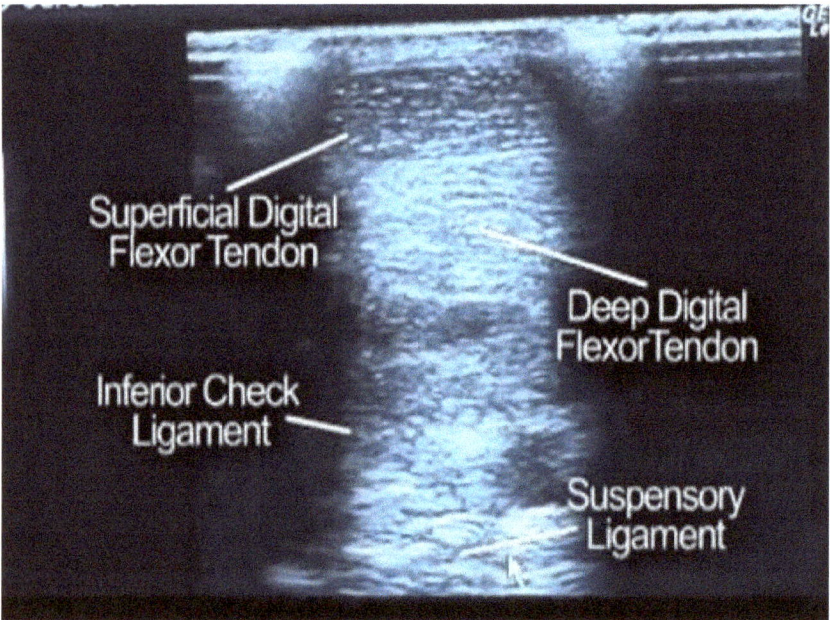

...... is best accomplished by ultrasound.

BOWED TENDON - TENDONITIS

Tendonitis- is irritation (inflammation) of a tendon.

Usually the tendons in the front leg are affected more often than the back legs

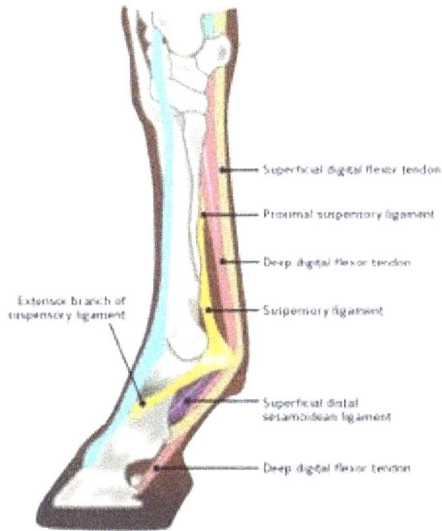

Tendons lay along the back of the legs and connect muscles in the legs to the bones in the ankle and foot. They are made up of strong fibers, but when stretched and worked beyond their strength, they tear and stretch. Tendonitis occurs with various degrees of the fiber disruption.

Tendonitis can be -

- acute – sudden and severe
- chronic – long standing and usually less severe

Tendinitis is most common in horses used at fast work, particularly racehorses, it is occasionally seen in jumping horses.

Signs include:

Severe lameness when the tendon is initially injured. The tendons are hot, painful, and swollen.

As the condition continues, there is fibrosis (scarring) with thickening and adhesions in the surrounding tendinous area. The horse with chronic tendinitis may be sound while walking or trotting, but lameness may recur under vigorous work.

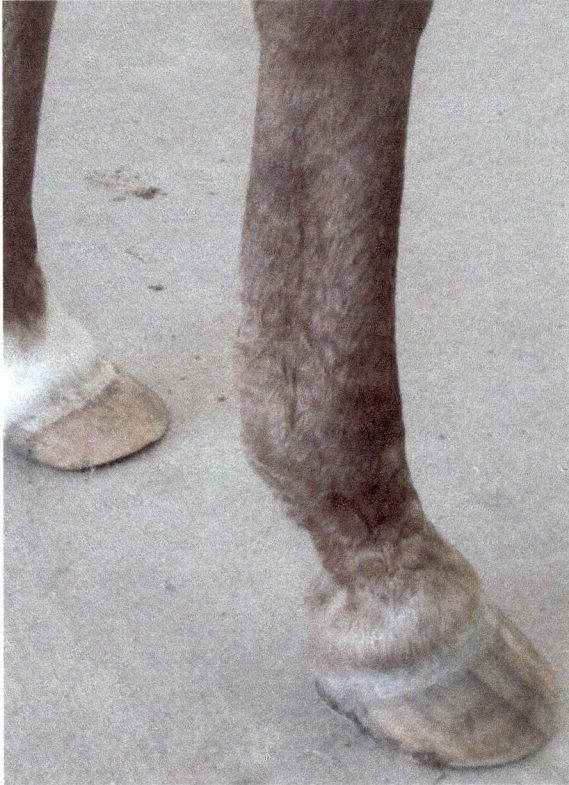

Ultrasound allows the veterinarian to determine the extent of the injury.

Seek veterinary care for tendon injuries.

CURB

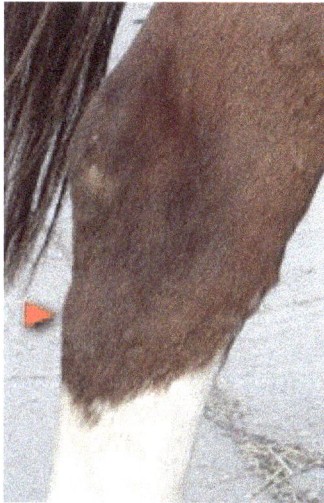

Curb is a term used to describe several soft-tissue injuries that cause swelling on the lower rear aspect of the rear leg under the hock.

Usually, the term "curb" is used to describe enlargement of the (long) plantar ligament on the rear (plantar) aspect of the calcaneus, but curb-like swelling may also be caused by tendinous-and ligamentous irritation from injury, superficial or deep digital flexor tendinitis, or a combination of injuries.

Curb is usually an injury of racehorses, particularly Standardbreds, and conformational abnormalities may predispose to curb.

Lameness varies from none to severe, depending on the structure involved and the extent of the injury.

Diagnosis and evaluation of the extent of the injury are confirmed by ultrasound.

Seek veterinary care for treatment recommendations.

CAPPED HOCK

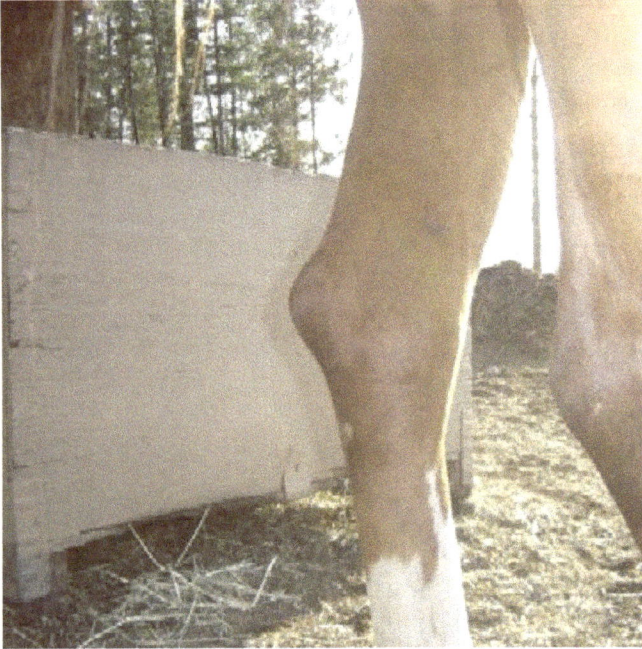

Capped hock is due to distention of the bursa (the membrane over the structures on the hock joint) or development of an acquired bursa over the point of the hock.

Capped hocks usually result from repetitive trauma (e.g., kicking or leaning on stable walls) and is not usually associated with lameness.

Occasionally, an abscess results if a penetrating injury occur. This may lead to painful swelling and lameness. Seek veterinary care for treatment recommendations.

Bone Spavin

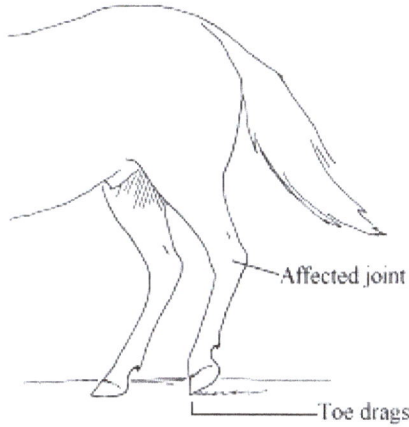

Figure 5

Bone spavin is arthritis in the joints of the hock.

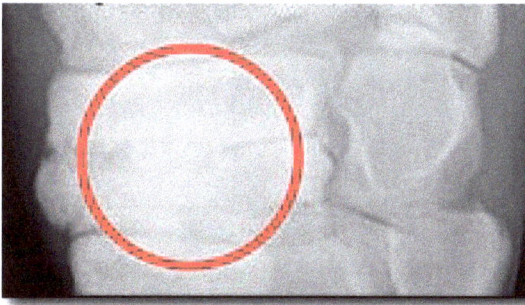

Lameness varies depending on the advancement of the arthritis and may be severe enough to end a horse's athletic career.

Bog Spavin

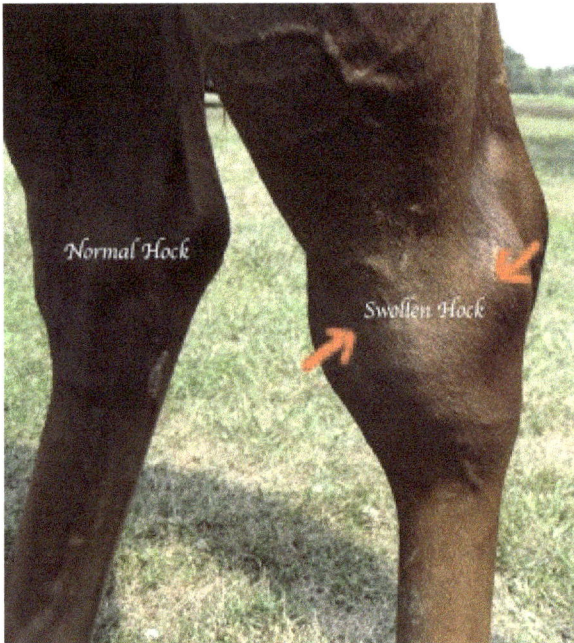

Bog spavin is a cosmetic swelling of the hock.

Swelling is due to fluid in the joint capsule of the hock joint.

This swelling is not accompanied by heat or pain, and it does not usually cause lameness.

In young horses, osteochondrosis must be considered. Seek veterinary care for evaluation of joint swelling.

BACK SORENESS

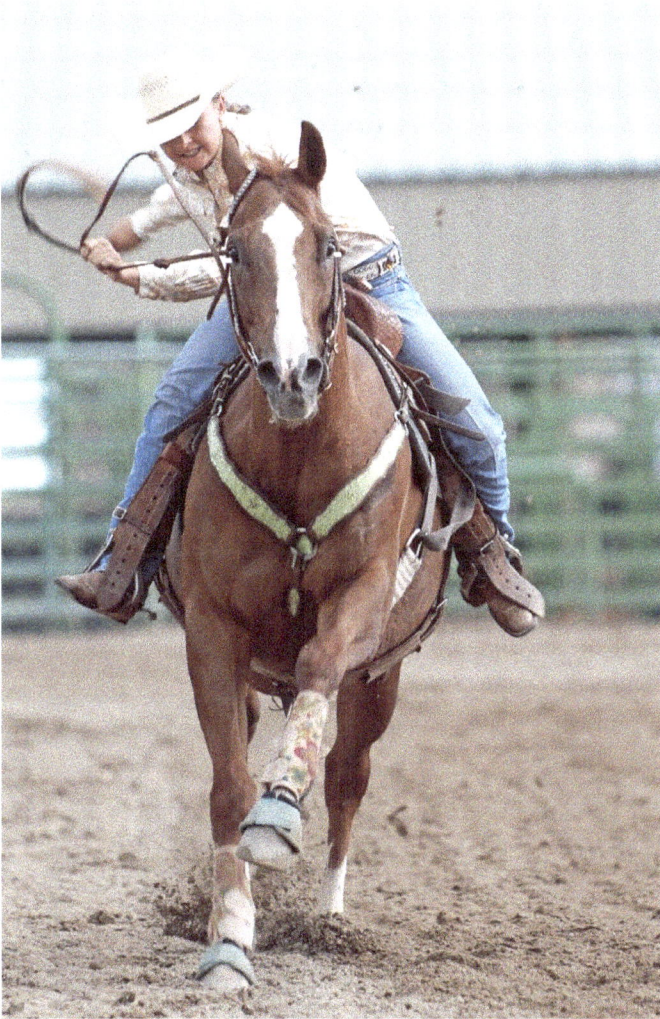

Overuse or damage to the muscles of the back are the most common causes of back soreness in horses.

Signs of back soreness include:

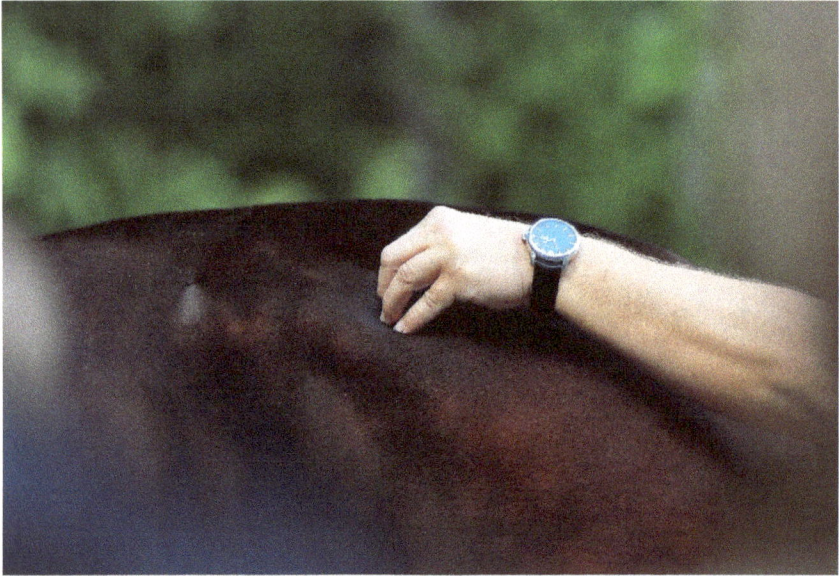

- soreness when touching the muscles along the back from the base of the neck to the tail
- crouching when the saddle or equipment is placed on the horse's back
- reluctance to stretch while working or bend while riding in circles
- sometimes lameness or a stiff gait may occur

Most of these injuries respond to rest and physiotherapy, although several weeks may be needed for full recovery.

EXERTIONAL MYOPATHY - TIE UP

Exertional myopathy (my-op-ah-thee)– is a disorder of the muscles where the muscle tension is so great the horse is in pain and has difficulty walking. Sometimes the horse is unable to walk at all.

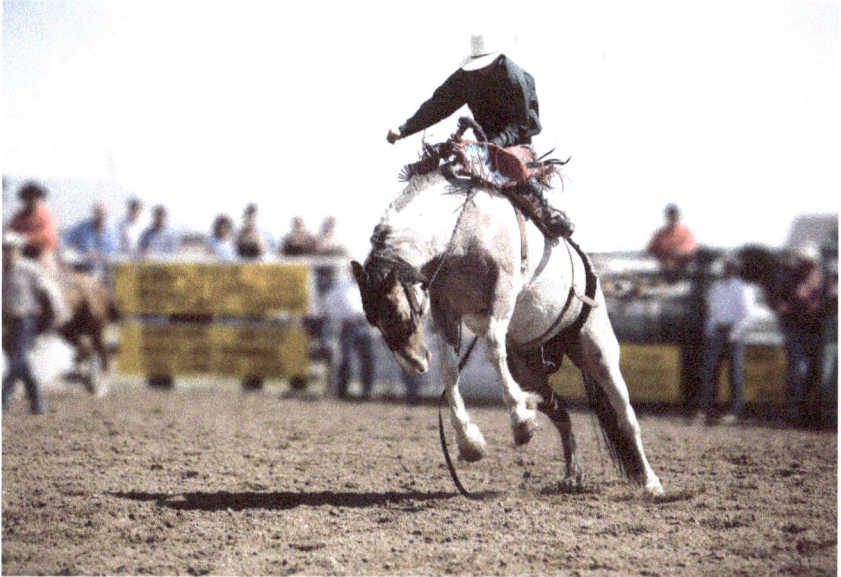

The cause of exertional myopathy is overuse or working an unfit horse too vigorously

When this occurs, there is damage to the muscle cells termed exertional rhabdomyolysis (rab- doe- my- oh- lie- sis).

Episodes range from mild to severe muscle injury- and the injury may lead to destruction or death of muscle cells.

It is damage to the muscles that causes:

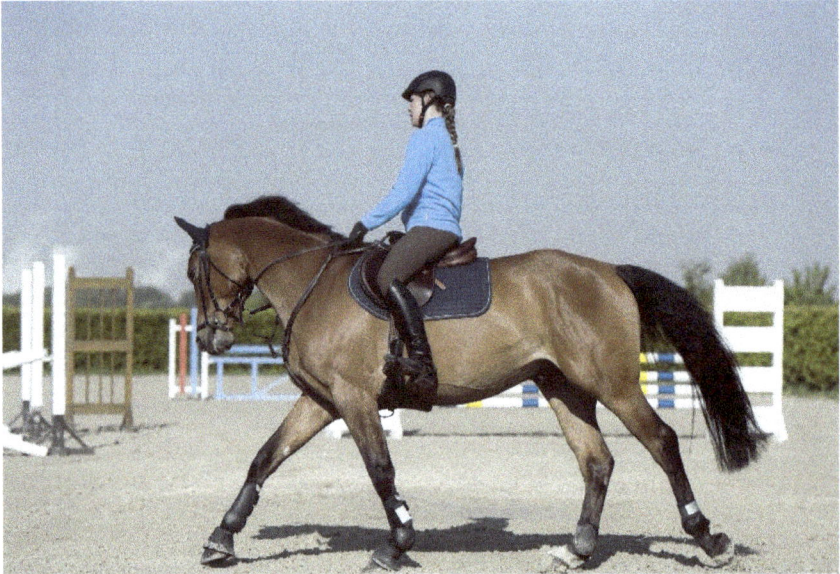

- excessive sweating – usually soon after exercise
- fast heart rate- an indication of pain
- fast breathing rate- an indication of pain
- reluctance or inability to move
- muscle flinching
- firm (hard) muscles to the back, rump, or back legs
- the horse may not be able to walk or get up
- in advanced cases, myoglobinemia occurs- myoglobin is the protein in muscle cells that attaches to oxygen – and, in myoglobinemia, the protein myoglobin is released into the blood
- this leads to myoglobinuria- myoglobin in the urine- which causes damage to the kidneys and kidney failure
- in severe cases the horse may be lost

Seek veterinary immediately if you have tie up syndrome.

Chapter 9

POISONS

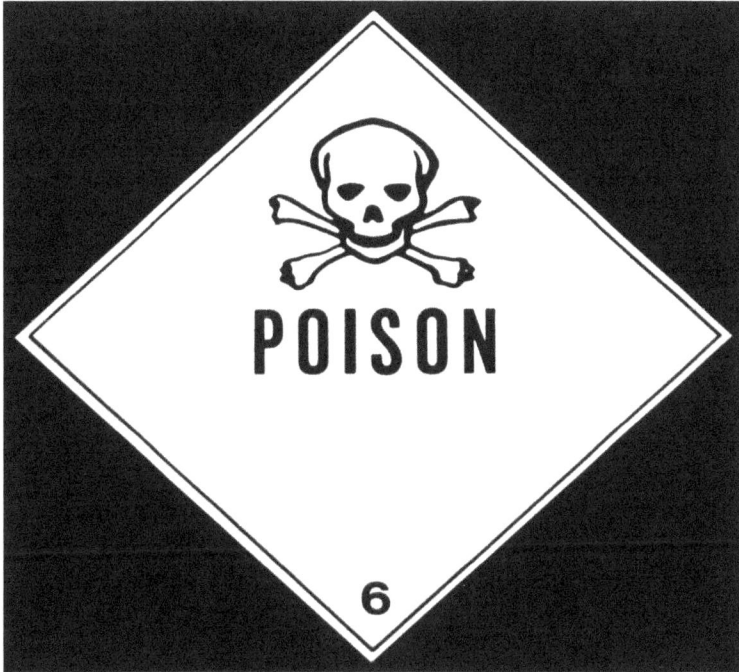

In most cases, it is difficult to determine the cause of poisoning in a horse because most toxic substances cause similar symptoms as well as can mimic other equine disorders.

Instead of trying to diagnose the horse, it is often easier to look around where the horse was stabled or roaming to attempt to spot any possible poisons.

Most of the time horses will not show an interest in poisonous plants or shrubs if the pasture they are grazing in is lush and adequate for their nutritional needs. It is still recommended to find poisonous forages and remove them from the pastures.

Although the symptoms caused by several types of poisons may be similar, treating them can differ, which is why it is important that, where possible, the poisonous substance is identified. If nothing can be found in the field, paddock or stable, then samples of the poisoned horse's feces, feed, stomach contents or body tissues may be analyzed.

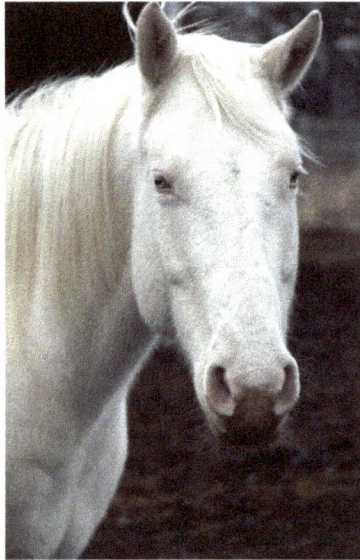

Common signs of poisoning in a horse include (but not limited to):

- loss of appetite
- uncoordinated movements
- lameness
- diarrhea – horses cannot vomit
- heavy or irregular breathing
- muscle twitching – and possible seizures
- dark colored or discolored urine
- drooling
- increased thirst
- jaundice – yellow color to the eyes, gums, and skin
- blindness and/or dilation of the pupils
- colic – abdominal pain
- swelling around the face, eyes or neck

Treating a Poisoned Horse

It is important to seek veterinary care immediately if you think a horse is poisoned because the longer a poison is in a horse, the less likely it will survive.

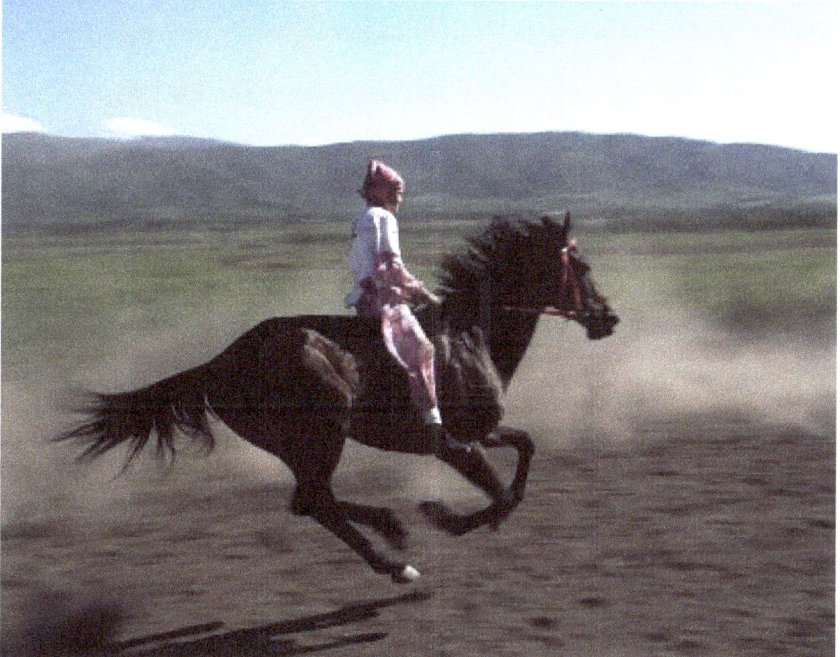

Of the many poisonous plants in the USA, only a few are potentially harmful to a horse.

The following pages have the 10 most poisonous plants for horses.

It is recommended to find any in and around the pastures your horses are in and remove them.

Tansy ragwort (*Senecio* spp.)

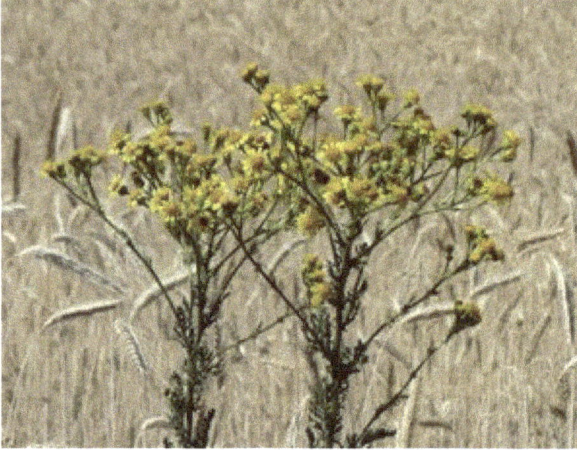

The danger with this poisonous foliage is that it contains chemicals that damage the liver of the horse. The damage to the liver is irreversible.

Signs of liver failure include:

- sensitivity to light
- decreased to no appetite
- weight loss
- signs progress to depression
- incoordination
- to jaundice – yellow coloring of the eyes, gums, and skin

There is no treatment for advanced liver disease.

Bracken fern *(Pteridum aquilinum*

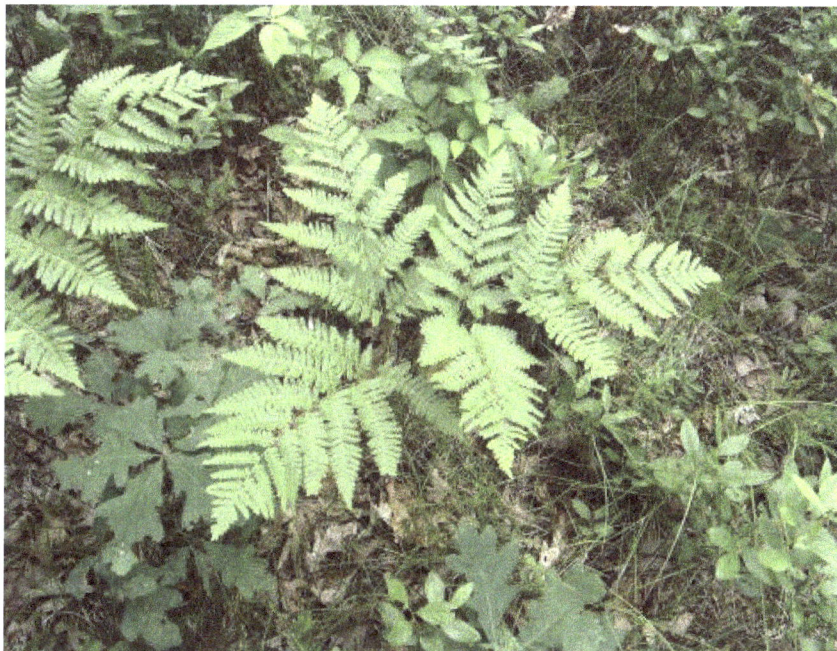

The danger with this poison is that it contains a chemical that stops a horse from absorbing thiamine- a vitamin B-1. Thiamine is necessary for proper nerve function.
.
Even though it may take a large amount of this to poison a horse, this is a unique poisonous plant because a horse may find it tasty and seek it out even if the pastures are adequate.

Signs of this poison are related to nerve dysfunction:

- depression
- incoordination
- blindness.

Hemlock *(Conium maculatum)*

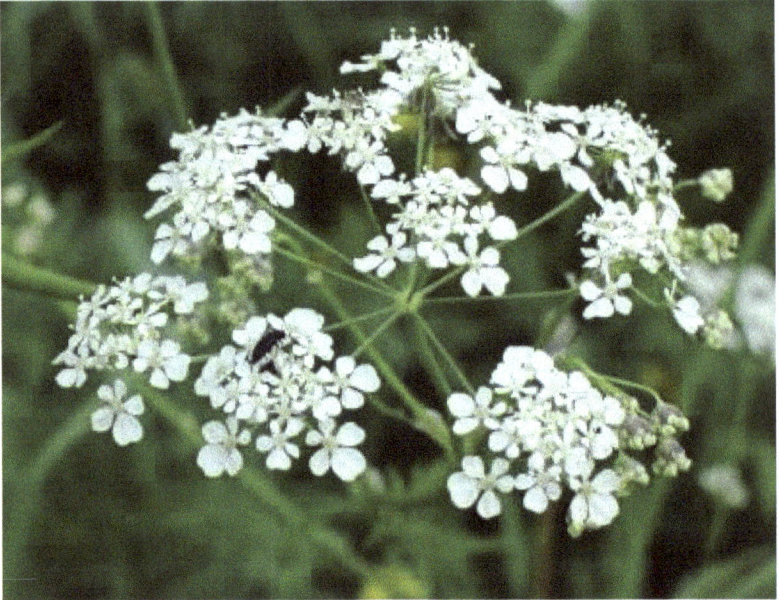

The danger with this poison is that, even though most animals will avoid the plant, small doses may be deadly.

Signs related to the brain and spinal cord may appear within 1-2 hours after ingestion and include:

- nervousness
- tremors and incoordination
- progressing to depression
- decreased heart rate and breathing rate
- to loss of the horse from breathing failure

There is no treatment, but if smaller doses were consumed, animals may recover with supportive care.

Johnsongrass/Sudan grass (*Sorghum* spp.)

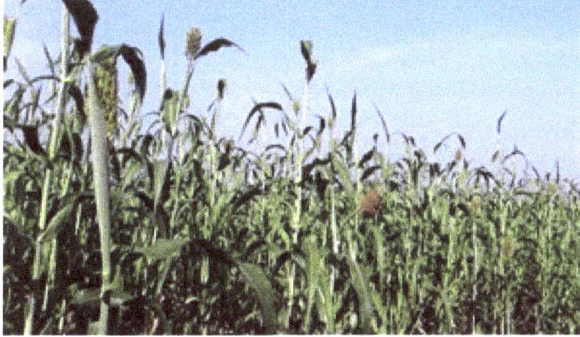

Both Johnsongrass and Sudan grass are grasses with wide, veined leaves that can grow to six feet in height. Both produce large, multibranched seed heads.

Signs of this poisoning include:

- signs consistent with cyanide poisoning
- fast breathing rate
- tremors
- frequent urination and defecation
- progressing to gasping for breath
- seizures
- loss of the pet

Locoweed (*Astragalus* spp. or *Oxytropis* spp.)

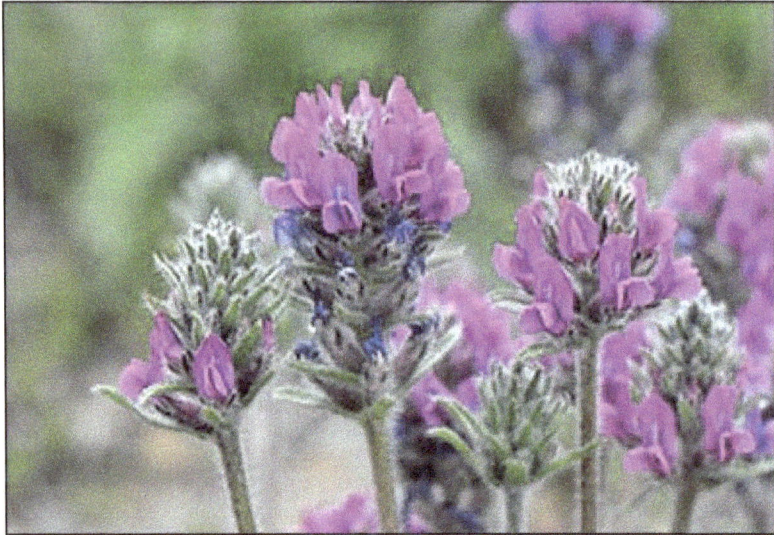

The danger with this poison is that these plants contain a chemical that inhibits the use of sugar in the brain.

Signs related to this poisoning include:

- bobbing of the head
- exaggerated high stepping gait or
- staggering
- they may fall

There is no treatment for advanced locoism, and its effects are irreversible. Horses with less severe poisoning may recover when access to the weed is removed.

Oleander *(Nerium oleander)*

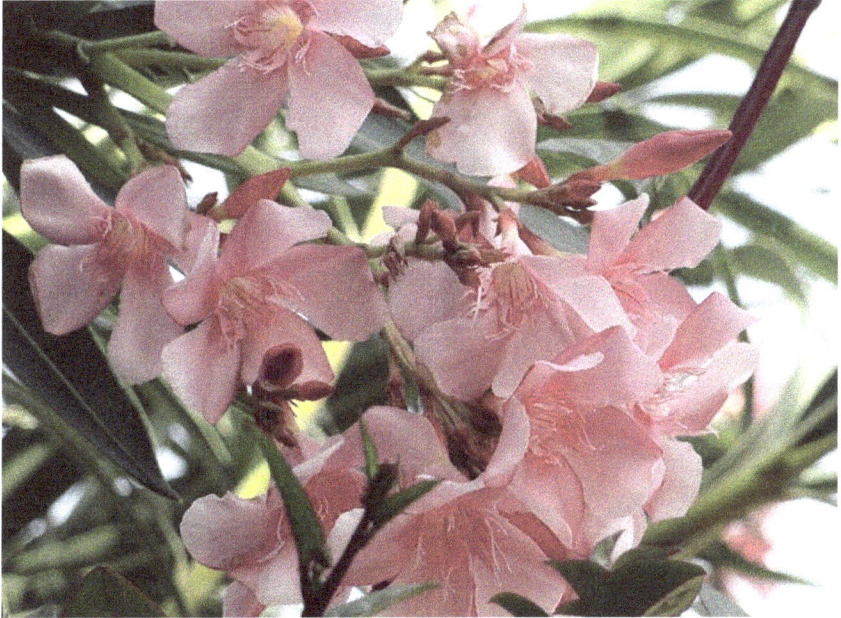

The danger with this poisonous plant is that all parts of the plant contain poisons that alter the heartbeat of the horse. The leaves are still poisonous when dried. As few as 30-40 leaves can cause loss of the horse.

Signs may be seen several hours after ingestion and last over 24 hours and include:

- colic – pain in the abdomen
- difficulty breathing
- tremors
- unable to get up when lying
- a slow OR fast heart rate may be seen

Red maple trees *(Acer rubrum)*

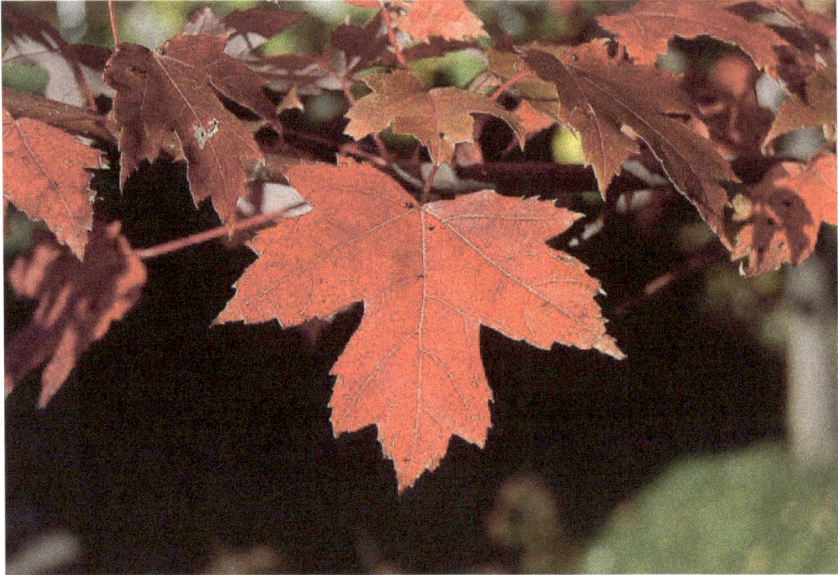

The danger is when these leaves wilt they become poisonous to horses. The poison causes red blood cells to break down. The red blood cells carry oxygen in the blood and cannot do so when injured. The liver and kidneys and other organs can also be damaged by this poison. Silver and Sugar Maples are also poisonous to horses.

Signs of poisoning can occur with a few hours and last 4-5 days and include:

- tiredness
- refusal to eat
- dark red- brown or black urine
- pale yellowish gums at first – then becoming dark muddy brown
- increased breathing rate and heart rate
- dehydration- loss of water

194

Water hemlock (*Cicuta* spp.)

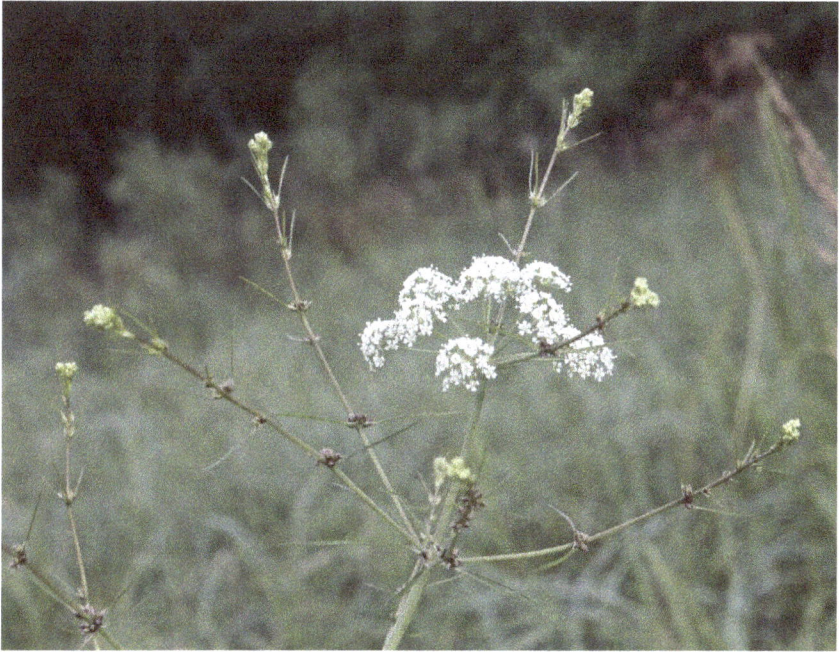

The danger with this poisonous plant is that it is considered one of the most poisonous plants in the USA. All parts of the plant contain a chemical that affects the brain and spinal cord. The root has the highest concentrations of the poison. Most animals avoid this plant.

Signs of poisoning may occur within 1 hour of ingestion and the horse may be lost in 2-3 hours- signs include:

- drooling
- dilated pupils
- nervousness
- progression to fast and difficult breathing
- degeneration of the heart and body muscles
- seizures
- loss of the horse

Yellow star thistle/Russian knapweed (*Centauria* spp.)

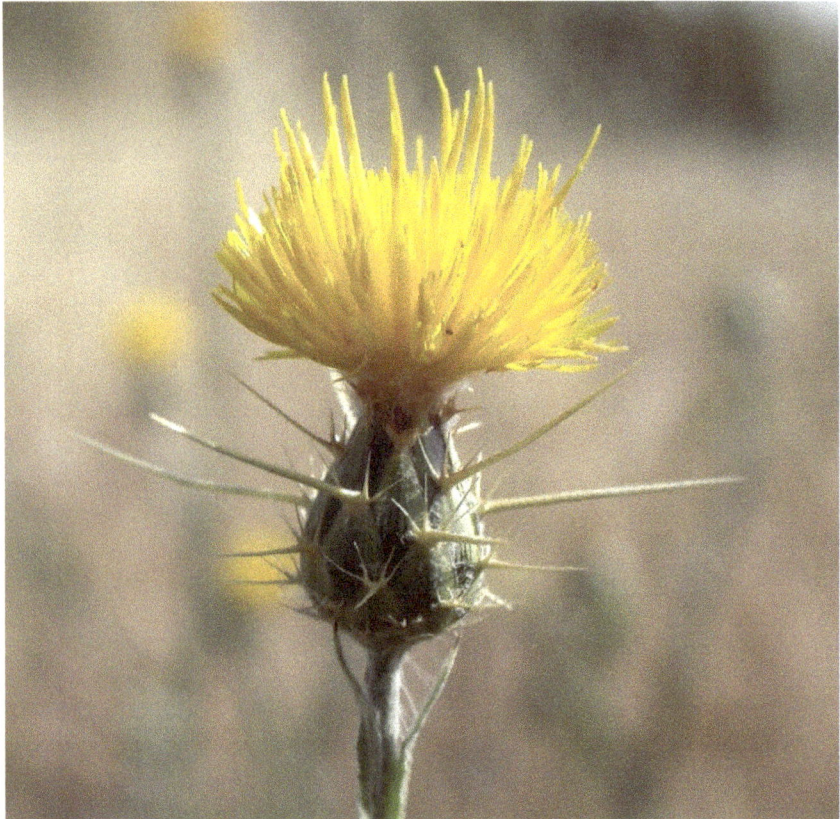

The danger with this plant is that it contains a chemical that inhibits the nerves that control the horse's chewing.

Signs include:

- tense or clenched muscles in the face and jaw
- the inability to chew or bite food
- weight loss

Yew (*Taxus* spp.)

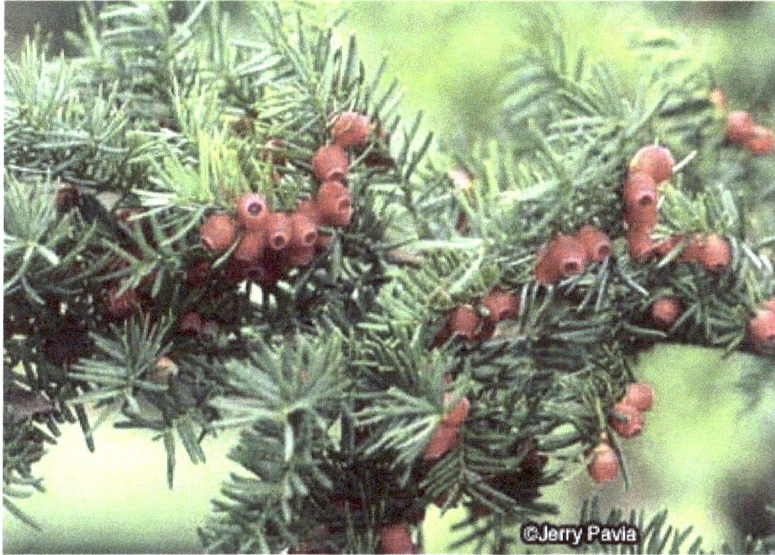

The danger is that all parts of the yew plant are toxic and cause the inability to breath. The toxin stops the horse's heart. The leaves are still toxic when dried. A single mouthful is deadly to a horse in minutes after being ingested.

.

Signs include:

- sudden death
- if alive, the horse may be shaking and colicky and have difficulty breathing and a slow heart rate.

.

There is no treatment for yew poisoning. Avoidance is critical; most yew poisonings occur when trimmings are thrown into a pasture after a pruning.

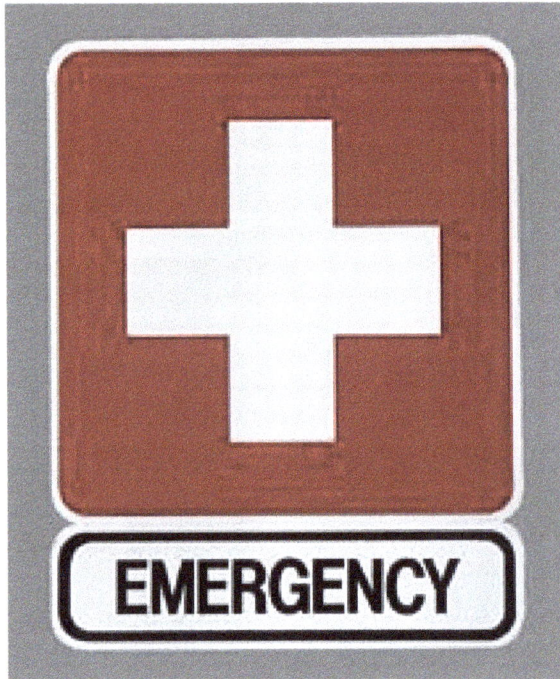

Many horse veterinarians are available for assistance if your horse requires care. Always seek help immediately. The quicker treatment is sought, the better chance a horse can survive a poisonous exposure.

Always have emergency phone numbers available – Veterinary Clinics and Poison Hotlines.

One Poison control number for horses is 888-426- 4435.

Chapter 10

Training

Horses can be the greatest fun ever, however, their size makes them potentially dangerous.

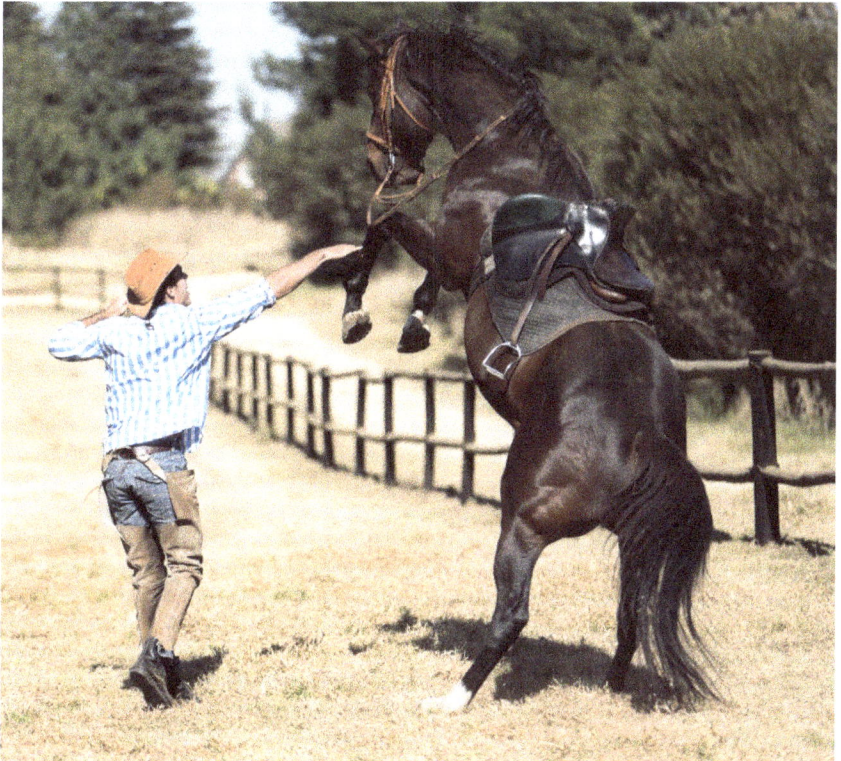

As much fun as horses can be, there are some bad habits- vices- that must be taken seriously.

Some vices include:

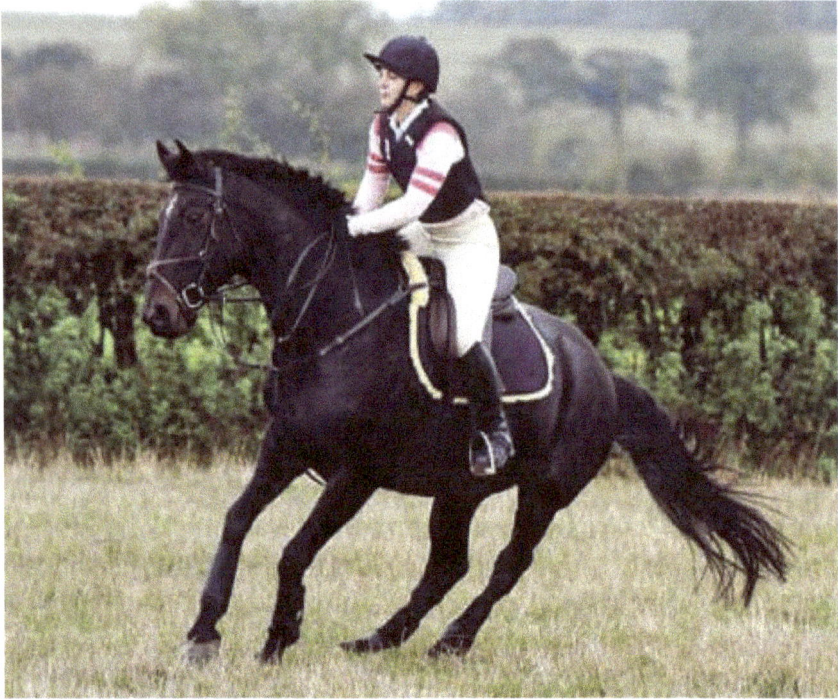

- balking – refusal to go forward- can be dangerous because it can lead to rearing or bucking
- barn sour – when a horse runs back to the barn- can be dangerous because the horse is typically out of control when they try to run back to the barn
- biting – sometimes horses bite when given treats by hand
- bolting- when turned loose- the horse turns, kicks and runs away in a dangerous manner
- head shy – makes it difficult to place a halter on the horse
- can't catch the horse

(more vices)

- the horse doesn't allow anyone to handle their feet
- halter pulling
- bucking

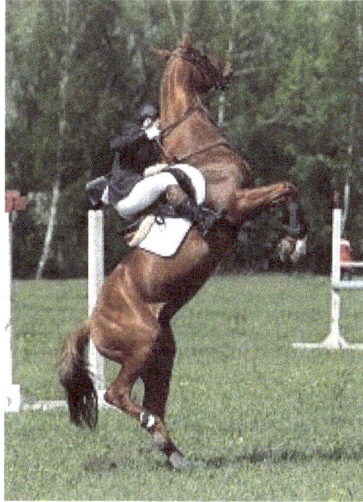

- rearing
- jigging- when the horse walks/trots with his/her head high and his back hollowed out under the rider
- kicking
- shying from objects
- striking
- tail wringing

(more vices)

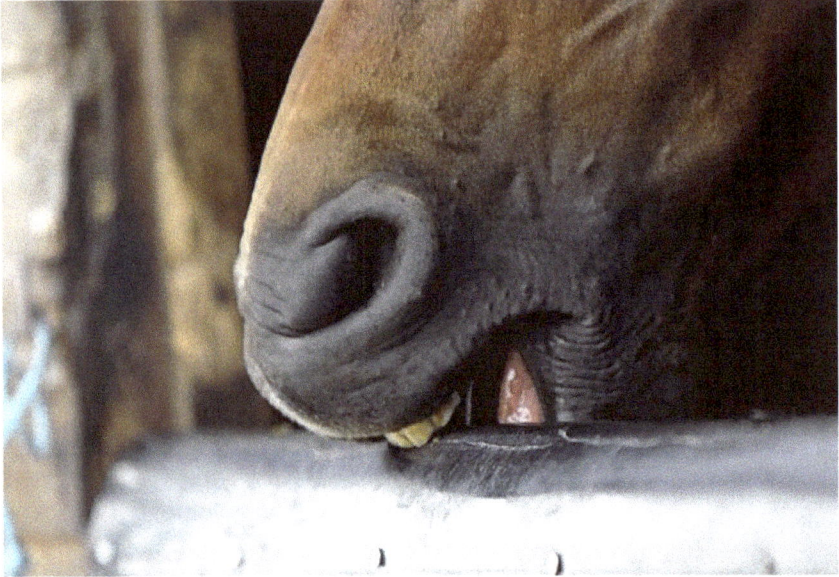

- cribbing
- wood chewing
- weaving
- stall kicking – can injure the horse or people in the stall
- pawing
- stalling walking
- coprophagy or dirt eating

- and throwing riders

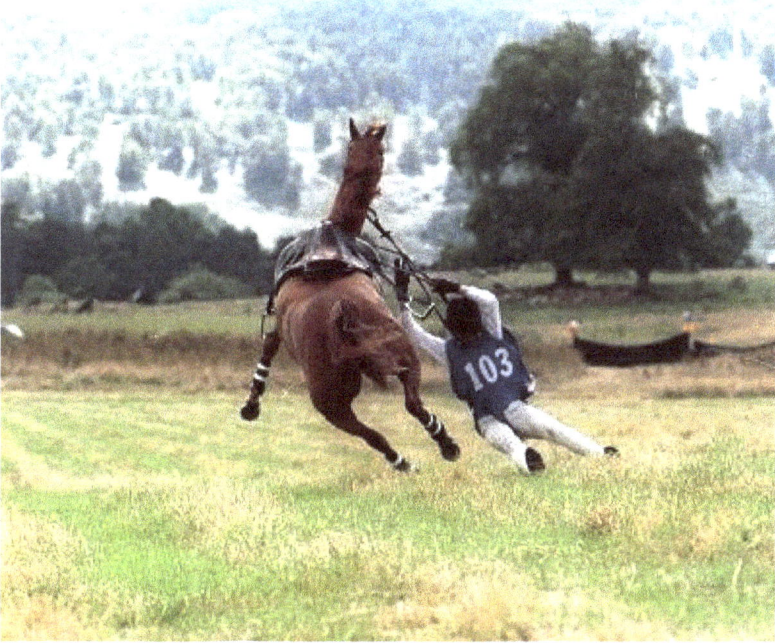

Bad habits- may require a professional trainer to help. You should always evaluate your skill level with a horse and their needs to make decisions that are safe. Consider the health of the horse and rider.

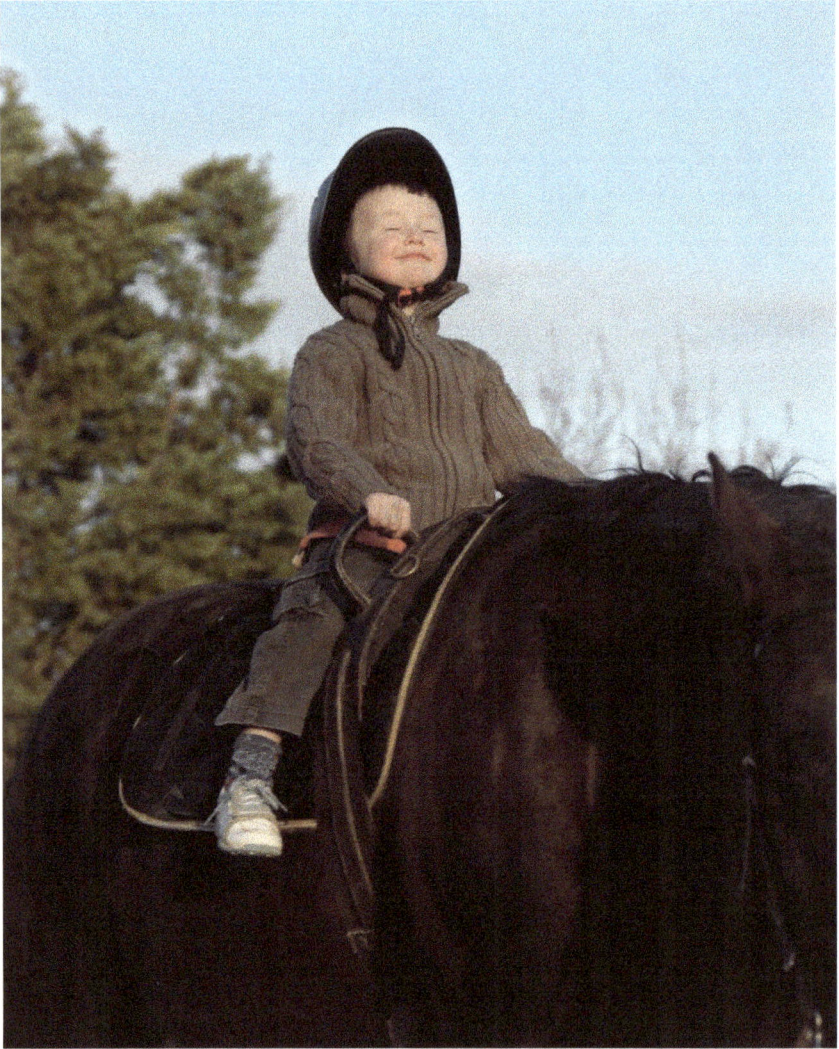

Child safe horses are recommended for children.

Some help for vices includes:

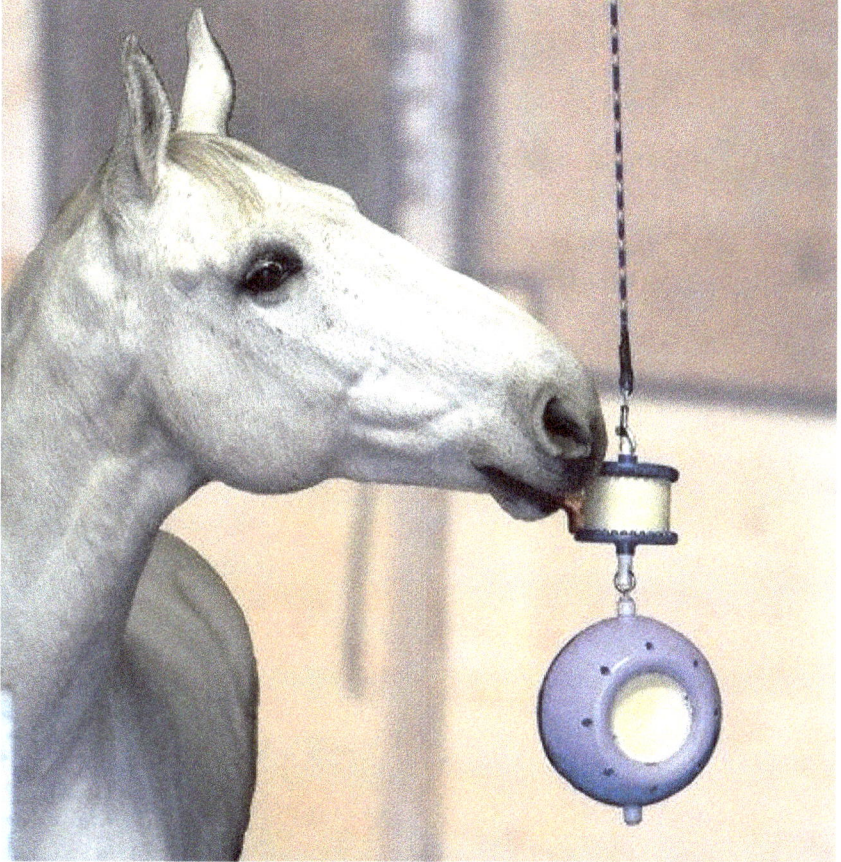

Consider a variety of toys available for horses who may be bored.

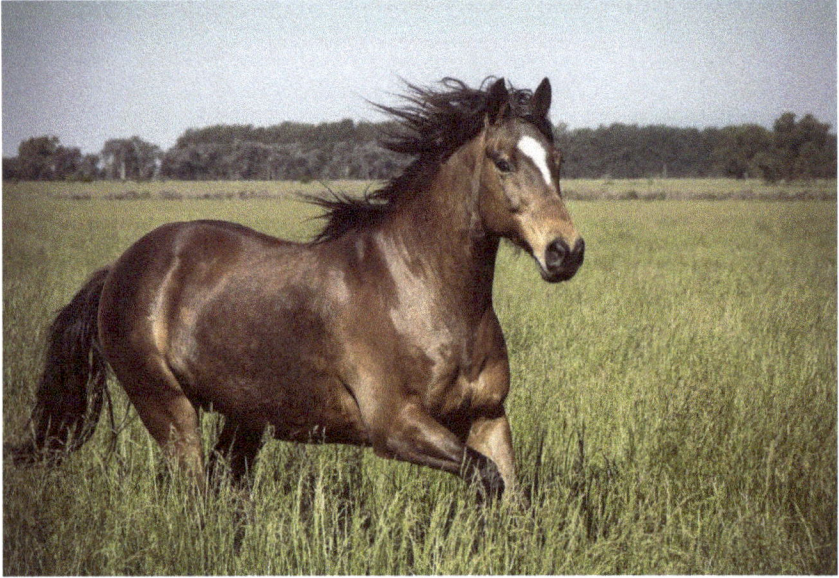

Turn out is also helpful for horses to run off excess energy.

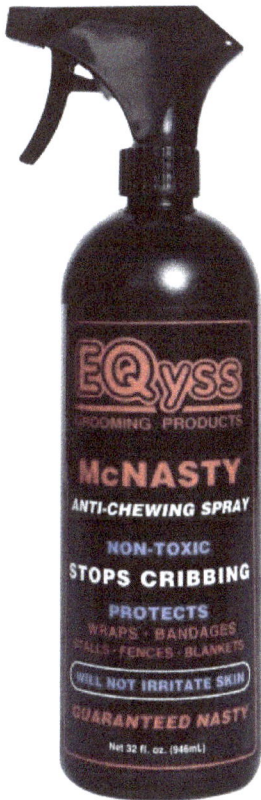

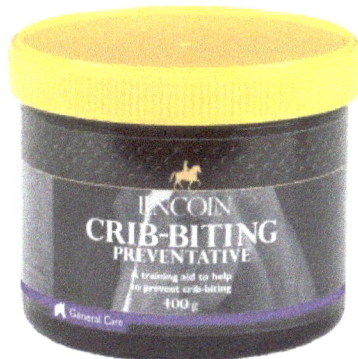

There are a variety of helpful products for several vices

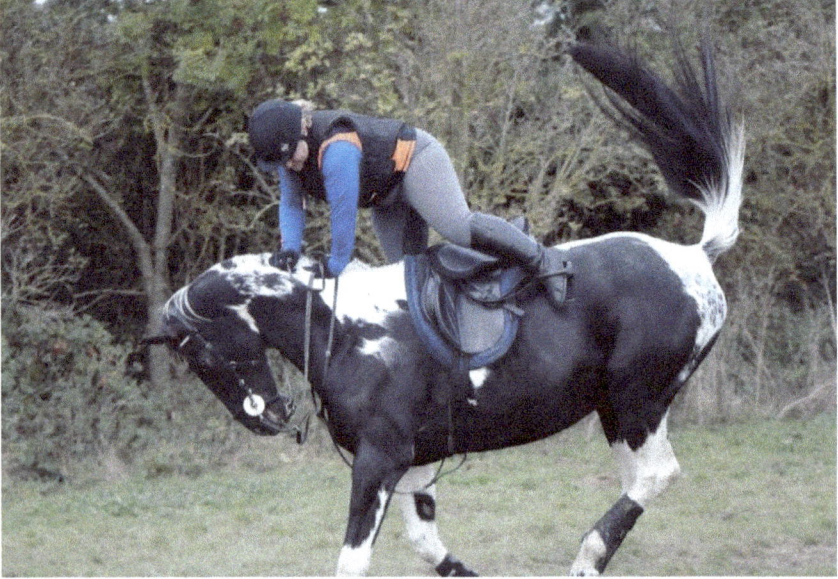

Remember to stay safe.

Chapter 11

Diagnostic Testing

A CLOSER LOOK

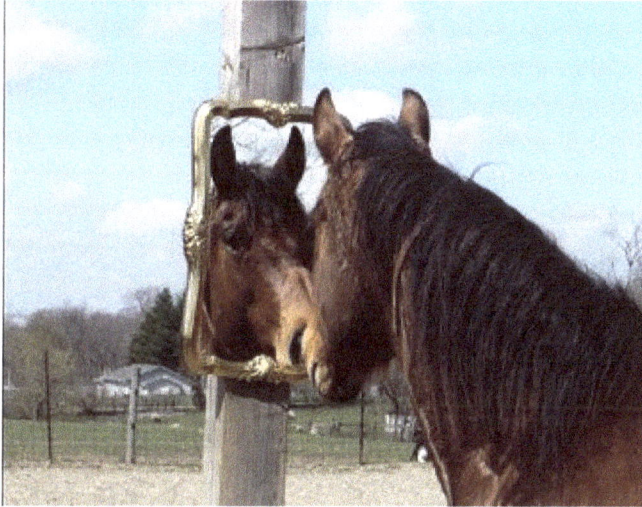

The first tool a veterinarian has to decide what disorders a horse may be experiencing is the physical exam.

The exam is important, however, does not provide all the necessary information to make decisions about disorders and care recommendations and a closer look is usually necessary.

Tests are available which help veterinarians make accurate decisions about disorders horses' experience- and therefore more accurate treatment recommendations.

Understanding the testing often recommended may be helpful to owners in making decisions regarding their horses' care.

Some common tests recommended and disorders are:

1. fecal samples (AKA poop samples)
2. blood tests to count cells
3. blood tests for screening body organs
4. measuring electrolytes
5. cushings in horses
6. ringworm
7. rain rot- rain scald
8. warts and papillomas
9. saddle sores
10. cancer of the skin
11. sarcoid
12. radiographs- x-rays
13. advanced testing- ultrasounds
14. eye disorders
15. and more

Poop Patrol

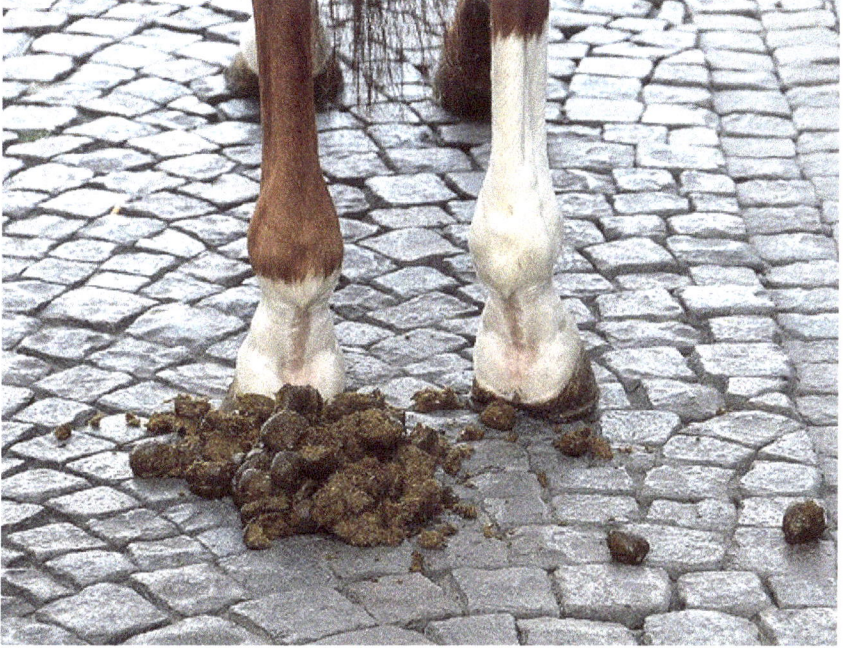

Examining horses' stool is critical to the health of every horse.

Intestinal parasites present a significant health threat for the life time of every horse.

Intestinal parasites -worms – can be silent thieves and killers because they can cause extensive damage without an owner realizing a horse is heavily infected.

Young and aged horses may be infected with parasites.

Regular deworming helps control parasites in horses.

Parasites are organisms that live part of their life cycle in a horse. They live in internal organs, body cavities and tissues, and take nutrients from the horse.

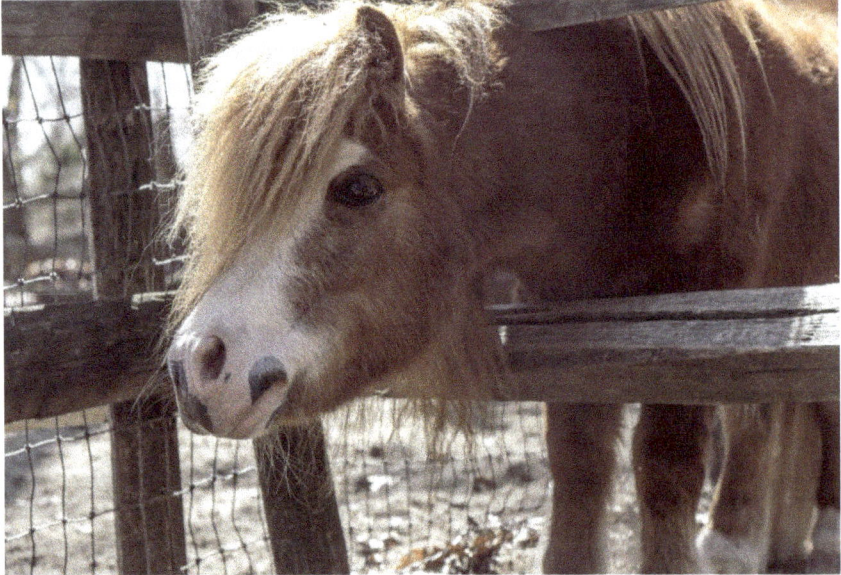

Part of a parasite's life cycle is in the environment, typically pastures. The horse is affected by many distinct species of parasites. The nature and extent of damage varies with the parasite and the number of parasites present. Parasites cost the horse and the horse owner in several ways:

- horses need more feed when infected with parasites
- parasites rob the horse of their nutrition/ nutrients
- parasites can cause anemia- a dwindling number of red blood cells that carry oxygen
- parasites cause young horses to grow slower and smaller
- parasites can interfere with a horse's reproductive or athletic abilities
- parasites may decrease a horse's immune system- making them more susceptible to other infections

212

Signs of Parasitism

The signs of parasite infection may include:

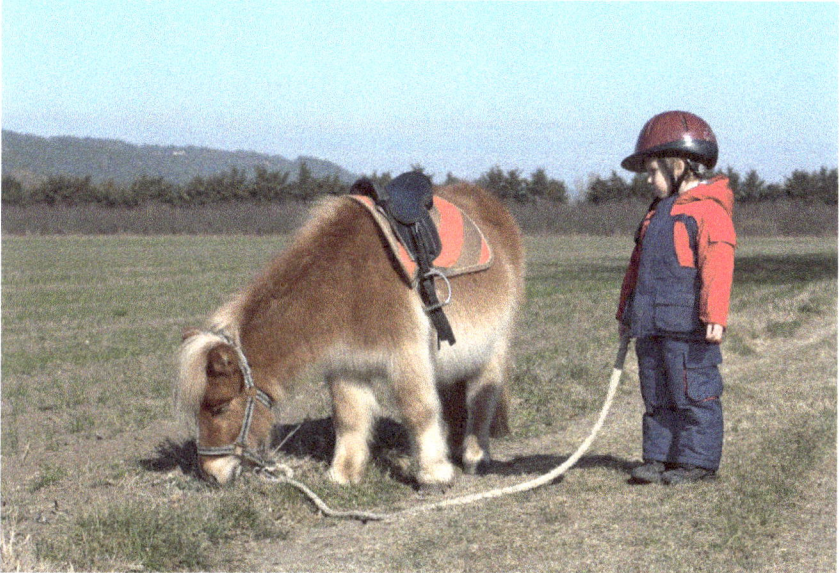

- weight loss

- dull, rough hair coat

- potbelly appearance

- decreased energy or tiredness

- coughing

- diarrhea

- colic – pain in the abdomen

- tail rubbing

More serious signs of internal parasites include:

- infection due to lowered resistance
- loss of valuable nutrition leading to un thriftiness
- permanent damage to the intestinal lining
- colic
- and even death

TYPES OF INTERNAL PARASITES

There are more than 150 species of internal parasites that can infect horses. The most common and troublesome include:

- small stronglyes (cyathostomins)
- roundworms (ascarids)
- tapeworms
- large strongyles (bloodworms or red worms)
- pinworms
- bots
- and others

The lifecycle of most internal parasites involves -

- eggs
- larvae (immature worms)
- and adults (mature worms).

Eggs or larvae are deposited onto the ground in the manure of an infected horse. They are swallowed while the horse is grazing, and the larvae mature into adults within the horse's digestive tract (stomach or intestines). With some species of parasite, the larvae migrate out of the horse's intestine into other tissues or organs before returning to the intestine and maturing into egg-laying adults.

Small Strongyles

Small strongyles are an important concern.

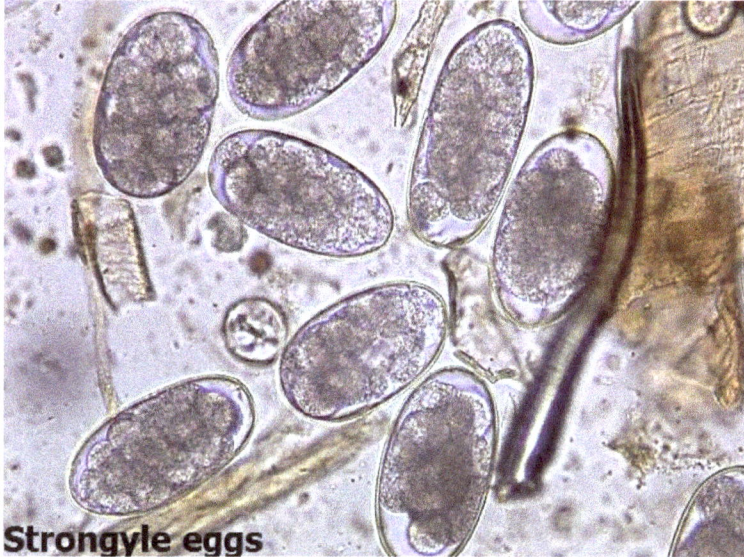

Strongyle eggs

Small strongyle larvae do not penetrate the intestinal wall or migrate through the tissues. They burrow into the lining of the intestine and can cause severe damage there, especially when large numbers of larvae emerge from an encysted stage all at once.

The large majority of horses tolerate small strongyles without showing signs of disease or discomfort, however signs may include:

- colic
- diarrhea in heavily infected horses
- weight loss
- slow and small growth in young horses
- poor conditioning
- decreased energy

Roundworms

Roundworms, (ascarids), are most often a problem in young horses - foals, weanlings and yearlings.

Adult roundworms are several inches long and almost the width of a pencil. Most foals do not show signs of roundworms, but, in large numbers, the roundworms can cause blockage (or impaction) of the intestine leading to colic

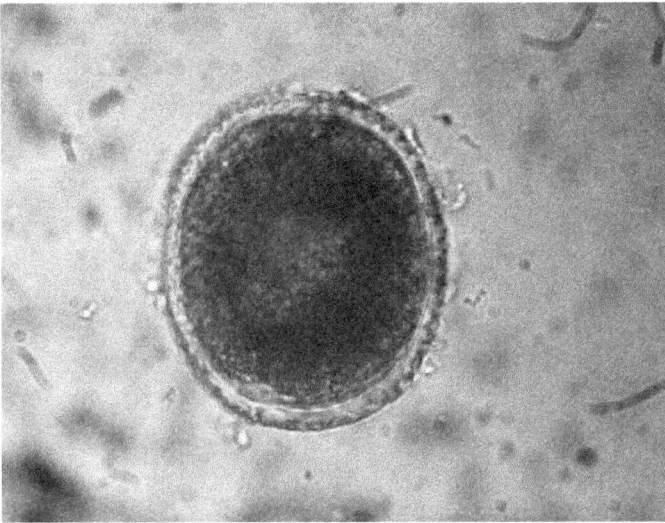

Roundworm infection in young horses can cause:

- coughing or infection including pneumonia– when migrating through the lungs
- liver damage
- damage to the blood vessels – especially ones to the intestines
- poor body condition and growth
- rough coat
- pot belly appearance
- slow and smaller growth in foals
- diarrhea
- and colic. – abdominal pain

Tapeworms

Like other parasites, many horses harbor tapeworm infections without showing any signs of disease or discomfort.

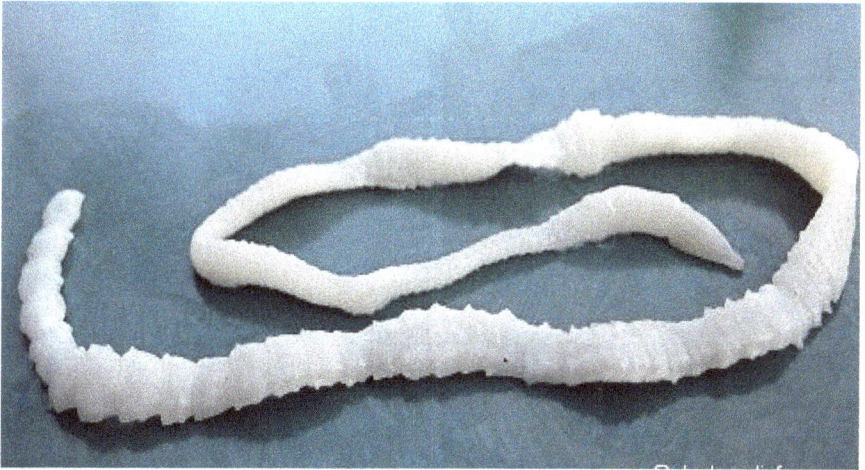

However, tapeworms can cause colic, ranging from mild cramping to severe colic that requires surgical treatment.

Tapeworms require and intermediate host- a host that the tapeworm grows in prior to growing in the horse. The horse tapeworm life cycle involves a tiny pasture mite as the intermediate host. Horses are at a risk of developing tapeworm infection when they eat this mite in the grass.

Large Strongyles

Large strongyles (bloodworms) have become extremely rare in managed horses because they are effectively controlled by most available dewormers.

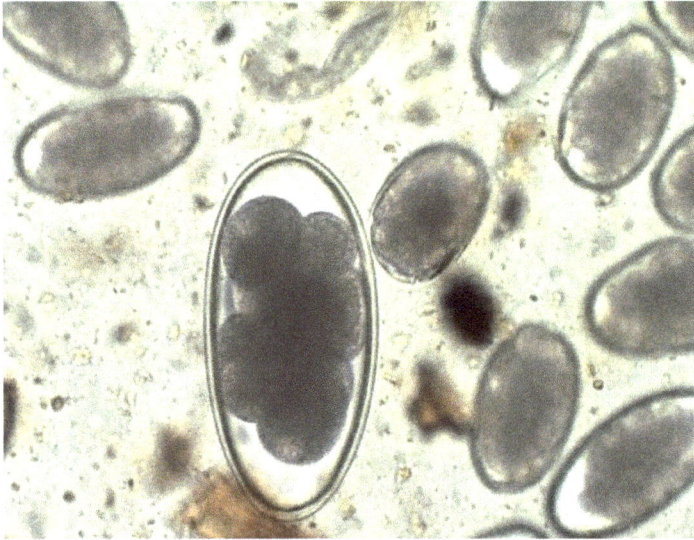

Infection with large strongyles can cause:

- unthrifty condition
- weight loss
- poor growth in young horses
- anemia (dwindling numbers of red blood cells that carry oxygen)
- and colic.

Pinworms

Pinworms lay their eggs on the skin around the horse's anus.

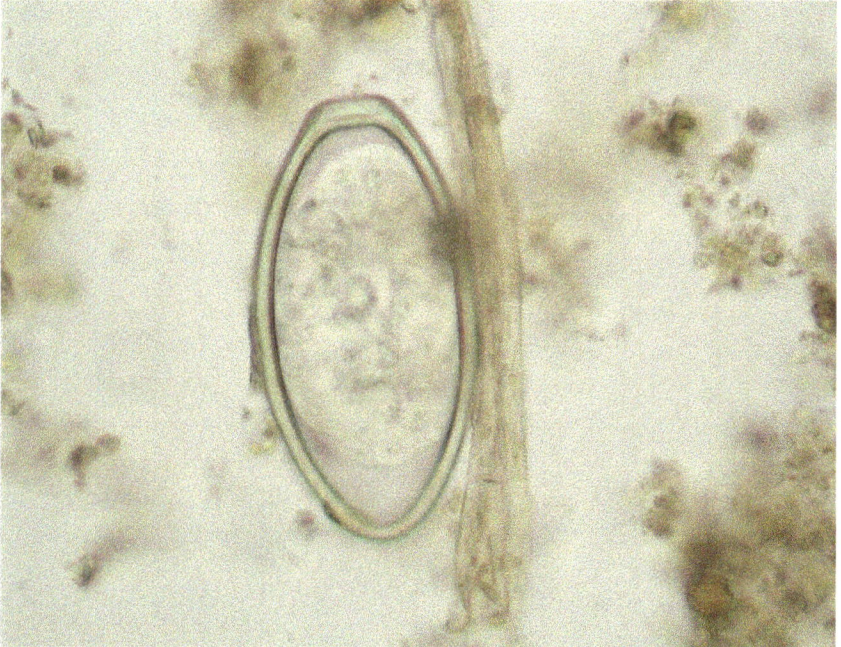

The irritation they cause makes the horse repeatedly rub its tail.

Bots

Bots are the larvae of the botfly and don't usually cause major health problems, although they can damage the lining of the stomach where they attach or ulcers in the mouth.

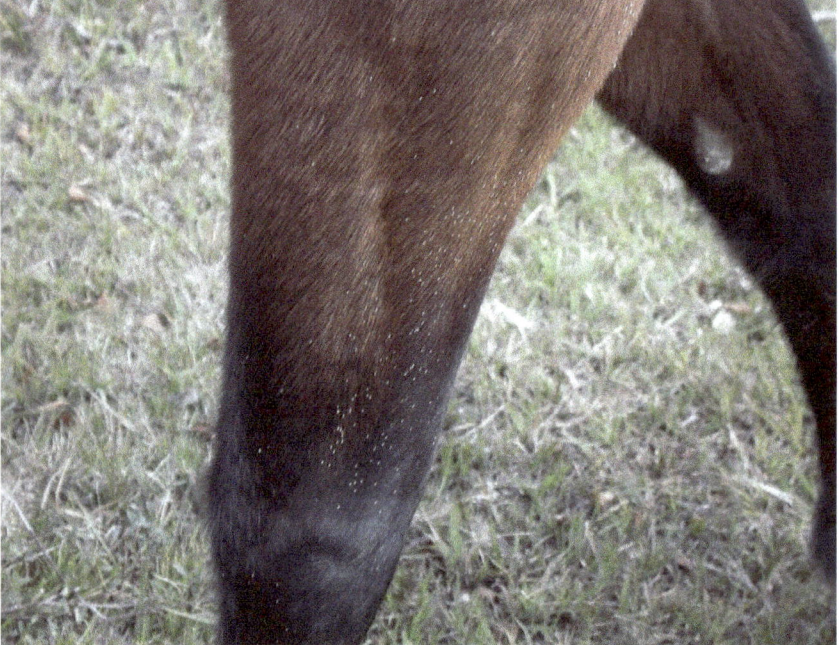

Three types of bots are:

- common horse bot (Gastrophilus intestinalis): the eggs are laid on the horse's body and ingested while self-grooming
- throat bot (Gastrophilus nasalis): the eggs are laid on the horse's neck and beneath jaw and the larvae make their way into horse's mouth
- nose bot (Gastrophilus haemorrhoidalis): is rare and the eggs are laid around the horse's lips

BLOODWORK

Veterinarians may recommend examining blood for the following:

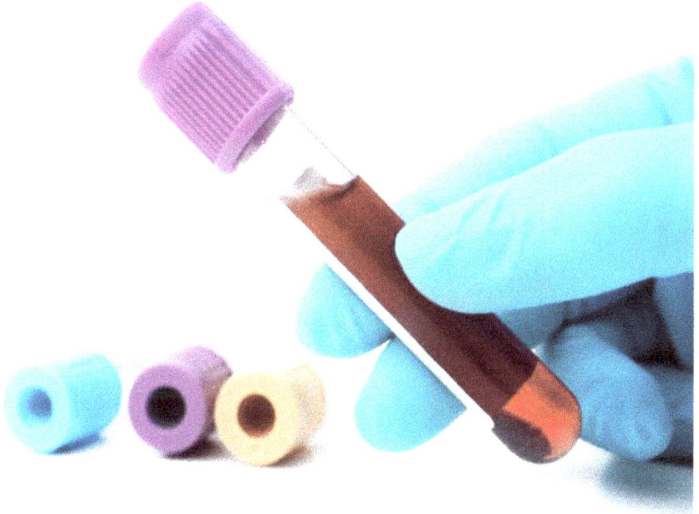

- complete blood counts- known as a CBC
- chemistry panels- also known as SMAC, internal organ function, chem- 7,12, 15
- electrolytes- including sodium, chloride, and potassium
- equine infectious anemia- EIA- discussed in chapter 2
- and others

Normal and Abnormal Values

Normal and abnormal test results have value to veterinarians in the care of horses.

When evaluating blood values, there are standards called 'normal' values. Health is when the values are 'normal' and disease may be identified when values are either too high or too low.

In addition, oftentimes, testing may be:

- conclusive- give enough information to conclude what is wrong with the horse
- suggestive - a disorder may be apparent, but need further testing to be certain
- inconclusive - some tests could indicate more than one disorder, so additional testing is necessary to be certain

Suggestive and inconclusive testing indicates a need for additional testing or referral to specialists for assistance with identifying disorders in horses.

FACTS ABOUT BLOOD

When blood is placed in a spinner and spun, it separates into 3 parts:

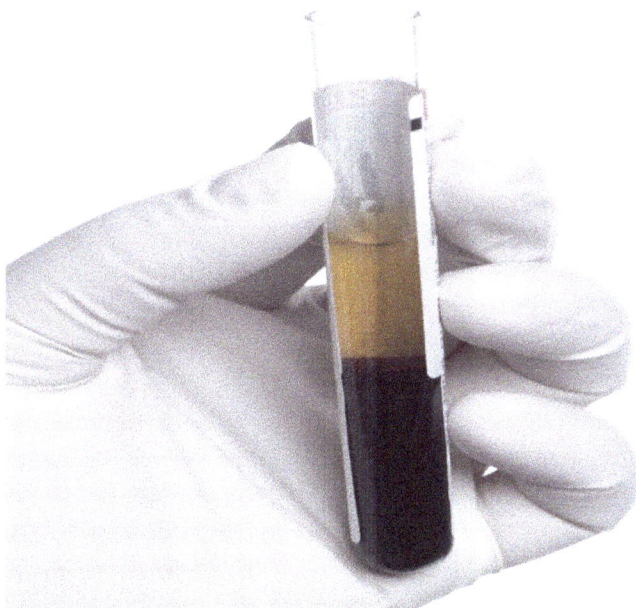

1. the liquid part that normally looks clear or slightly straw colored
2. the red blood cells – which settle to the bottom
3. the white blood cells - a small layer of cells which are usually in the layer between the liquid part and the red blood cell

These parts of the blood are tested.

CBC- the complete blood count

The cells counted are:

1. the red cells- which carry oxygen in the blood
2. the platelets- which help with blood clotting
3. the white blood cells- there are several types which help protect horses by fighting infection - and other functions (such as fighting cancer)

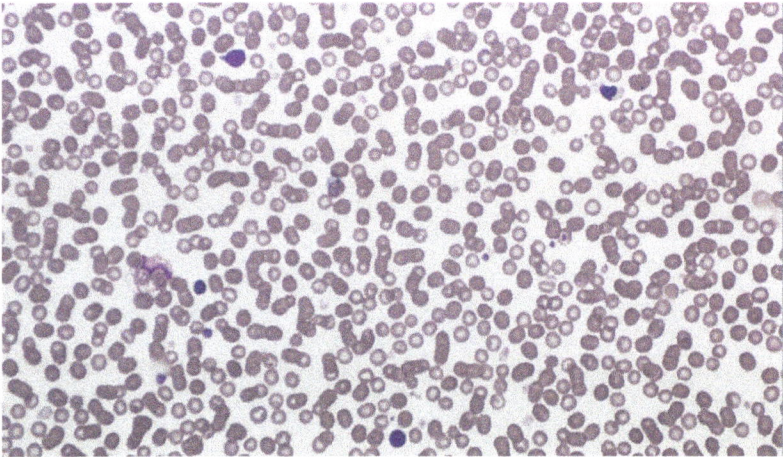

Veterinarians gain information when cell counts are:

- too high
- too low
- or just right (normal)

With this information, the veterinarian can create treatment plans for the care of horses.

CHEMISTRY

"Chemistry" tests are performed on the liquid part of blood and screen different items.

SODIUM   21
POTASSIUM   16
CHLORIDE   1.04
CARBON DIOXIDE   15
UREA NITROGEN   6.1
CREATININE   3.0
BUN/CREATININE RATIO   9.7
URIC ACID
PHOSPHORUS   64
CALCIUM   3.7
CHOLESTEROL, TOTAL
HDL CHOLESTEROL
CHOLESTEROL/HDL RATIO
LDL CHOL, CALCULATED   112
See footnote 1   7.6
TRIGLYCERIDES   8
PROTEIN, TOTAL

Some items relate to blood levels reflecting organ health such as liver and kidney health, and some values relate to sugar in the blood, calcium, and even cholesterol. When these screening values are not within a 'normal' range, illness is usually indicated as well as the need for treatment and/or further testing or referral to specialists to decide what disorders may be present.

Several different chemistry 'panels' are available – the number associated with the chemistry panel usually indicates how many items are being tested – for example-

Chem 6- tests 6 basic items in the blood
Chem 12- tests 12 items
Chem 25- tests 25 items

And so on.....
It is easy to see that the more items tested for, the more information is obtained.

Specific Tests for Chemistry Evaluation

As with the CBC- there are 'normal' standards established for the chemistry items tested for. Values that are 'too high' or 'too low' may indicate a need for treatment

Some 'chemistry' items tested are:

- Glucose - AKA – the blood sugar
- Creatinine- screens for kidney health
- BUN- the 'blood urea nitrogen' -screens for kidney health
- ALT- (alanine aminotransferase)- screens for liver health
- AST- (aspartate aminotransferase) -screens for liver health
- GGT- (gamma glutamyl transferase) screens for liver health
- Albumin- is a protein found in the blood
- Globulins- are proteins found in the blood
- Alkaline Phosphatase - screens for liver and/or muscle and bone health
- Cholesterol- measures the amount of cholesterol in the pet's body
- Total bilirubin- screens for liver and gall bladder and red blood cell health
- Phosphorus- measures the level of phosphorous in the pet's blood
- Amylase – screens for pancreatic health
- Lipase- screens for pancreatic health
- CK- creatine kinase- an enzyme related to muscles

ELECTROLYTES

Electrolytes are dissolved chemicals with electrical charge found in the liquid part of the blood. Electrolytes are important for the health of the horse and are involved in many aspects of body function-including the heart, and muscle, and nerve action.

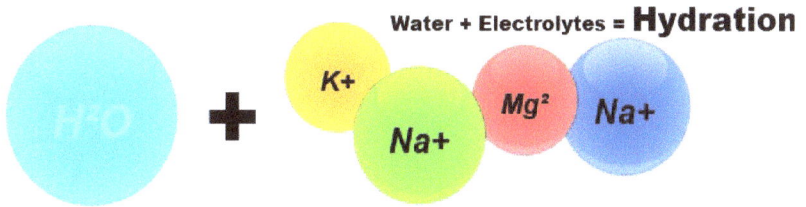

Water + Electrolytes = **Hydration**

H_2O + K+ Na+ Mg^2 Na+

Some electrolytes are:

- sodium
- chloride
- potassium
- calcium
- magnesium
- and others

CUSHINGS IN HORSES

Cushiings is also known as Pituitary Pars Intermedia Dysfunction or PPID. Cushing's Disease is a dysfunction of the pituitary gland- a gland found in the brain.

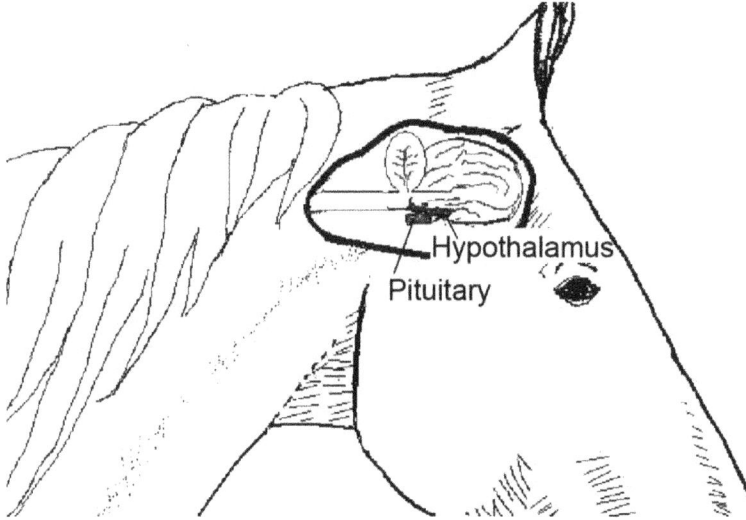

Equine Cushing's occurs when a tumor called a pituitary adenoma develops in the pituitary gland. As this tumor slowly grows, it sends chemicals called hormones to the adrenal glands- 2 glands that are located over the kidneys. This causes the adrenal glands to make excessive cortisol hormone.

The disease can be confirmed by blood tests. Cushings cannot be cured, but effective treatment can improve a horse or pony's' quality of life.

228

Cushings is most common in older horses -18 - 23 years old - but has been seen in horses as young as seven.

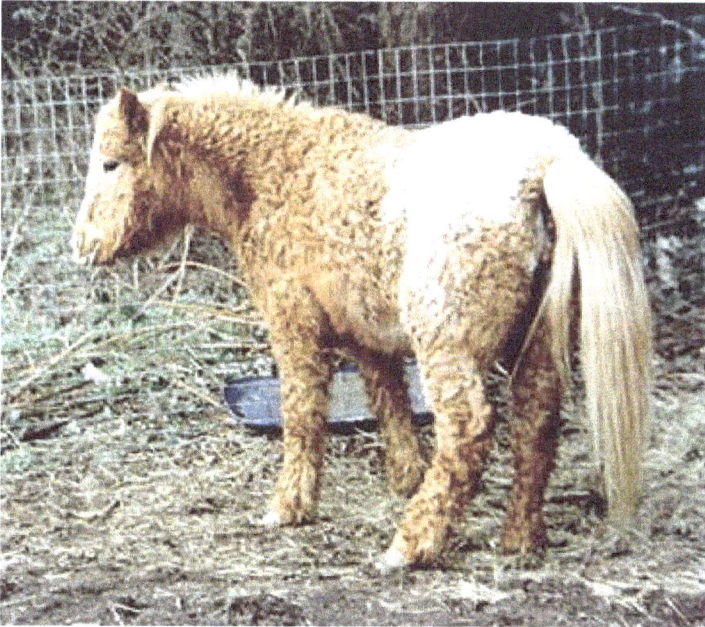

Signs of Cushings include:

- hypertrichosis (long, curly hair that DOES NOT SHED)
- decreased muscling along top line and rounded or pot-bellied appearance
- sluggish and listless expression
- fat deposits, especially along the crest of the neck and over the tail head
- laminitis
- increased drinking and urination
- recurrent infections
- abnormal sweating
- absent reproductive cycle/infertility

SKIN DISORDERS

RINGWORM

Ringworm is an infection of the skin by a fungal organism – of the *Trichophyton* or *Microsporum* families.

Rounded hairless patches with crusty, scabby skin are the usual signs of ringworm.

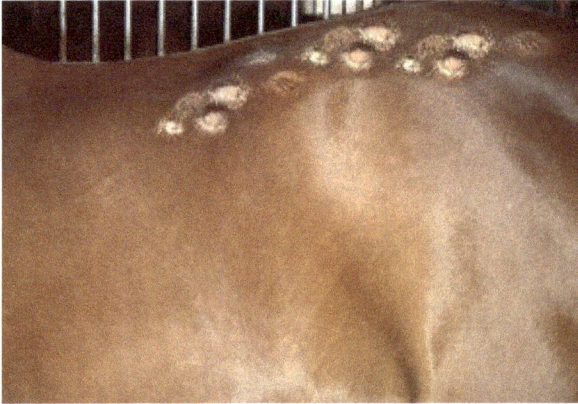

It is recommended to keep separate tack, equipment, and grooming supplies for every horse.

Quarantine new horses brought to the farm for at least two weeks to make sure they aren't carrying ringworm or other contagious diseases.

If an outbreak occurs, clean and disinfect any tack or equipment as well as wash stalls and fences that infected animals have had contact with. Remember people can get ringworm as well as all other animals, including cats and dogs. Always wear gloves when handling infected horses and exposed equipment.

RAIN ROT- (Rain scald)

Rain scald is a bacterial infection of the skin with *Dermatophilus congolensis* bacteria that resides on the skin without causing infection unless there is a heavy hair coat or moist environment.

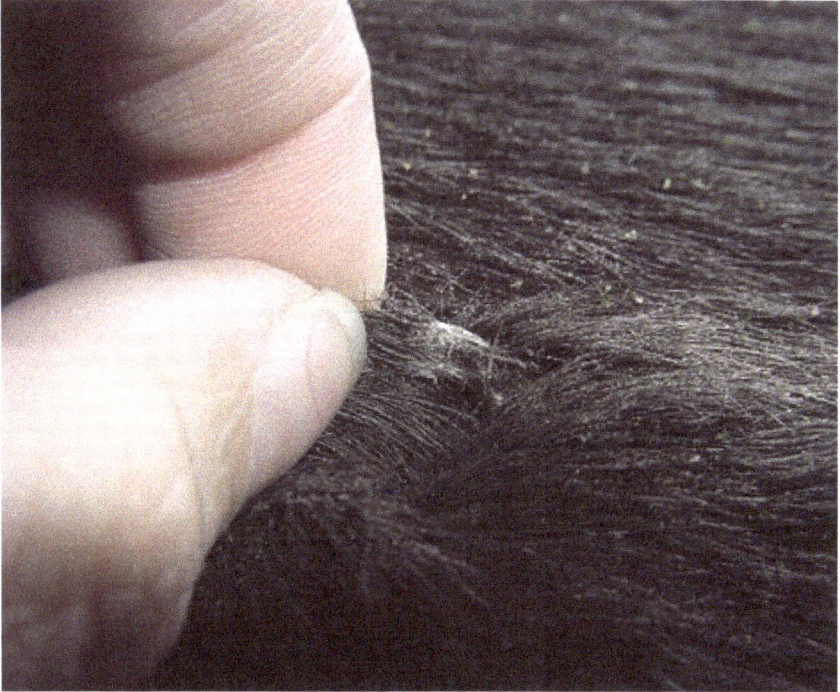

Signs include scabby crusts that form raised bumps with upright tufts of matted hair. The crusts often form along the topline and where rain runs down the barrel, shoulders or hindquarters, but also on the lower legs or faces of horses who regularly stand in mud or graze in tall, wet grass. Over time, the crusts peel off, leaving small, round bare spots. Pus may also be seen under newly sloughed scabs.

To prevent rain scald, provide dry areas that turned-out horses can retreat to in wet weather. Waterproof blankets and light sheets may also help keep pastured horses dry. Groom often.

Disinfect all blankets and equipment that contacted an infected horse before reuse.

WARTS/PAPILLOMAS

Warts and papillomas are caused by the equine papilloma virus and appear in the skin as small raised masses. They may be a single mass or many and are seen around the eyes and muzzle, but can be seen anywhere – including the ears and genitals and lower legs.

The growths do not cause pain and are harmless.

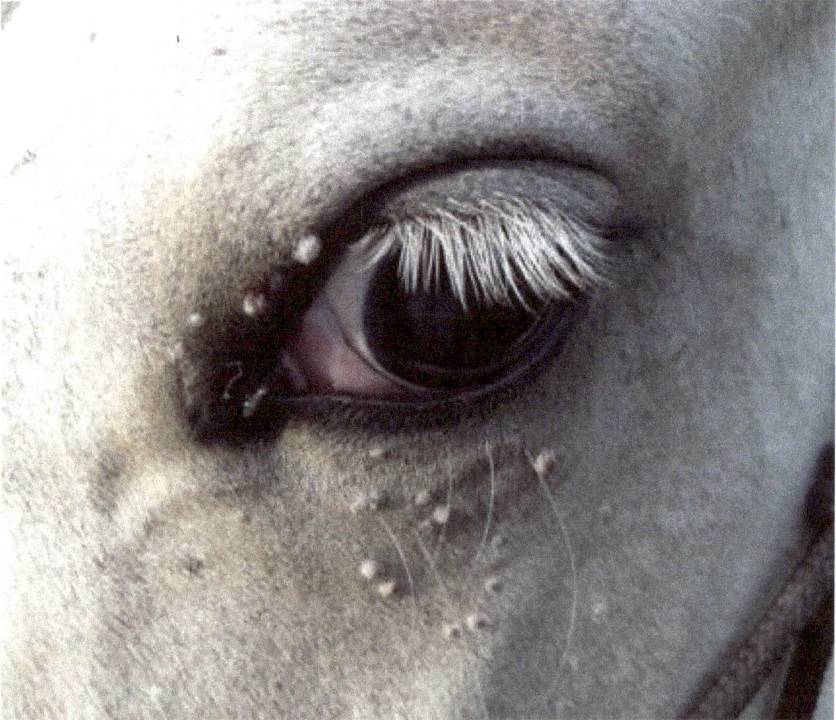

Most warts, if left alone, shrink and disappear, leaving no scars.

They usually disappear more quickly in younger horses than older horses. If a wart is interfering with equipment, or an owner would like them removed, consult a veterinarian.

SADDLE SORES

Saddle sores (galls) are a condition of skin injury under the pressure areas of tack. The areas of skin under the saddle on riding horses and on the shoulder area of driving horses are the sites of skin and soft tissue injury. Clinical signs will vary, depending on the depth of injury as well as any complications from secondary infections.

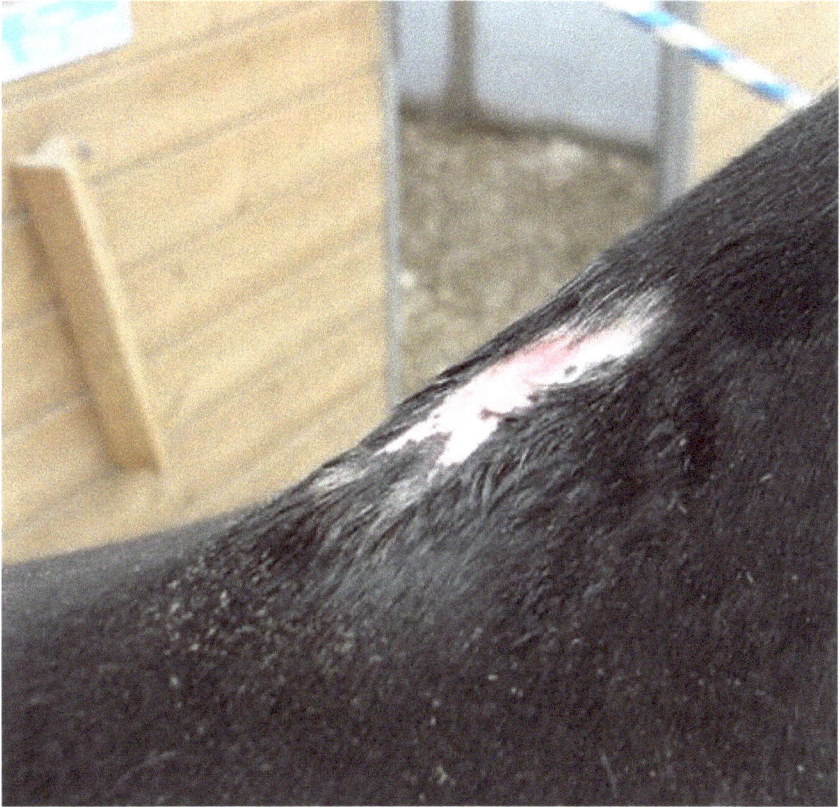

The cause of saddle sores is ill-fitting tack. When the condition occurs, the treatment is absolute rest of the affected parts.

CANCER OF THE SKIN

Melanoma – is a pigmented cancer in the skin. It is cancer of the melanocytes in the skin.

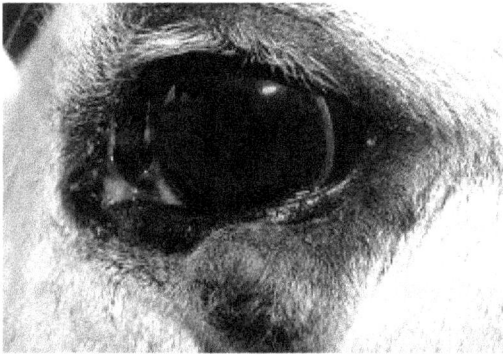

In horses, melanoma appears to be more prevalent in gray horses because of the dark skin pigmentation. While some forms of skin cancer are benign (harmless), melanoma is often malignant (harmful cancer that spreads to other body areas).

Melanoma can occur on the face, genital area, rectal area, or any area of the body of the horse. Some masses can be quite large.

SARCOID

Sarcoid – a tumor found on the skin of horses, donkeys, and mules.

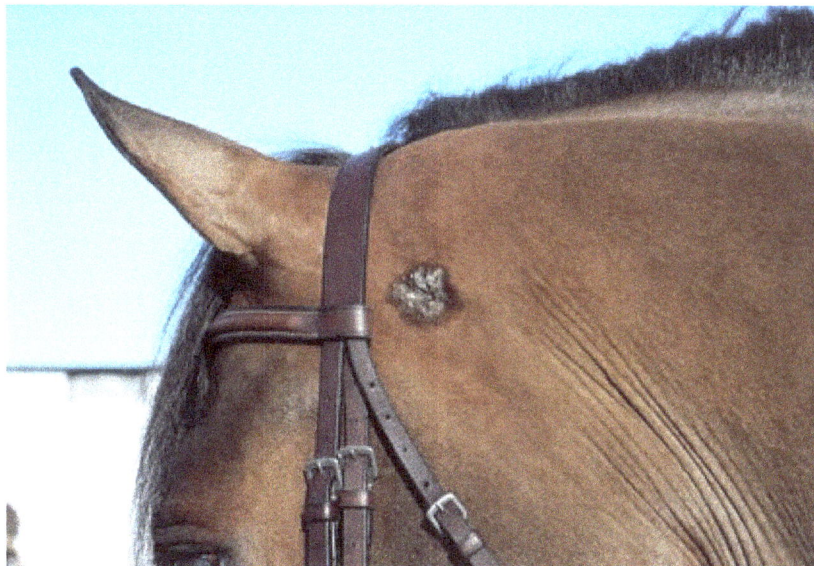

Sarcoids are one of the most common skin neoplasia (cancers) seen in horses.

Sarcoids are generally benign (harmless) but can be locally invasive to deeper and more extensive tissue.

XRAYS

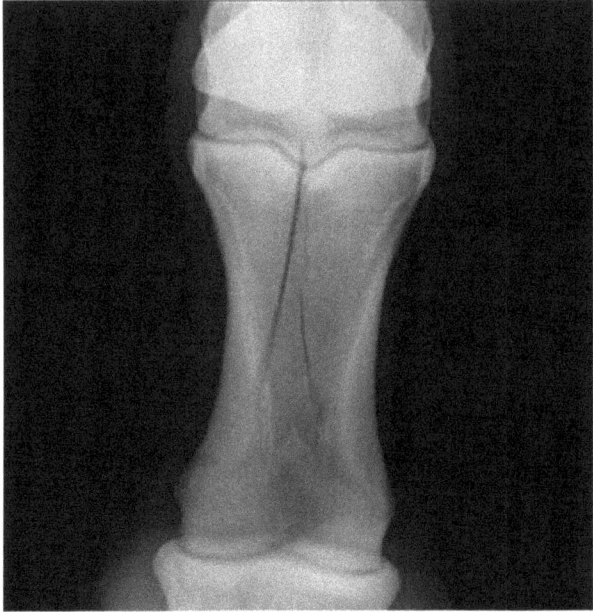

Radiographs- AKA- x-rays- are mainly useful in identifying broken bones and arthritis. In the horse, the chest and abdomen are quite large and may be difficult to x-ray, however, some larger clinics are able to x-ray the heart and lungs of horses. Ponies, miniature horses, and foals are easier to x-ray all parts of the body for evaluation – such as the intestines, internal organs, lung infection, and more.

ULTRASOUND

Ultrasound is a noninvasive test without radiation available for more detailed imaging of body organs such as the heart, liver, kidneys, pancreas, eyes, lymph nodes, testicles, ovaries and uterus, pregnancy and foal health in mares, intestines, spleen, stones in bladders, and pregnancy as below.

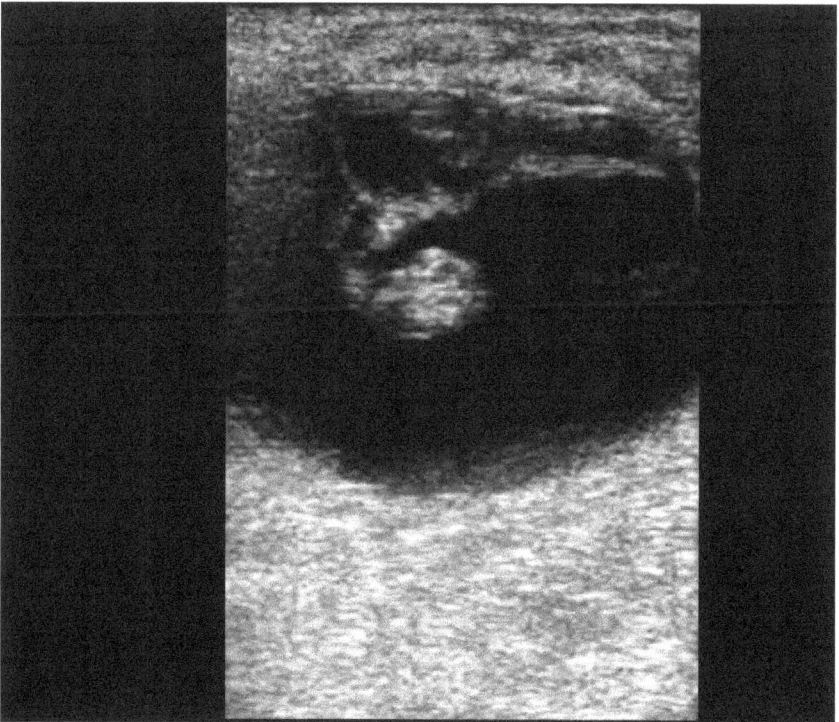

Some veterinarians are skilled at this technique while some veterinarians advise referral to specialists for this testing

EYES

The horse has the largest eyeball of any land mammal.

The horse's eye magnifies everything he sees larger than a human eye does.

Horses have excellent peripheral vision and can see almost 360 degrees around him or her.

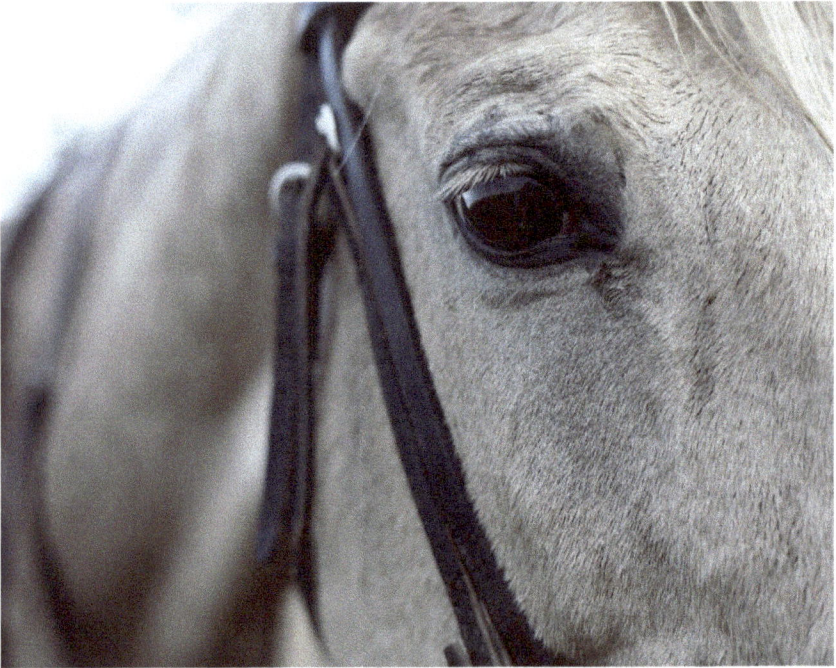

Some disorders of the eye include:
- corneal ulcers
- foreign bodies
- eyelid laceration
- uveitis
- and more

Corneal ulcers

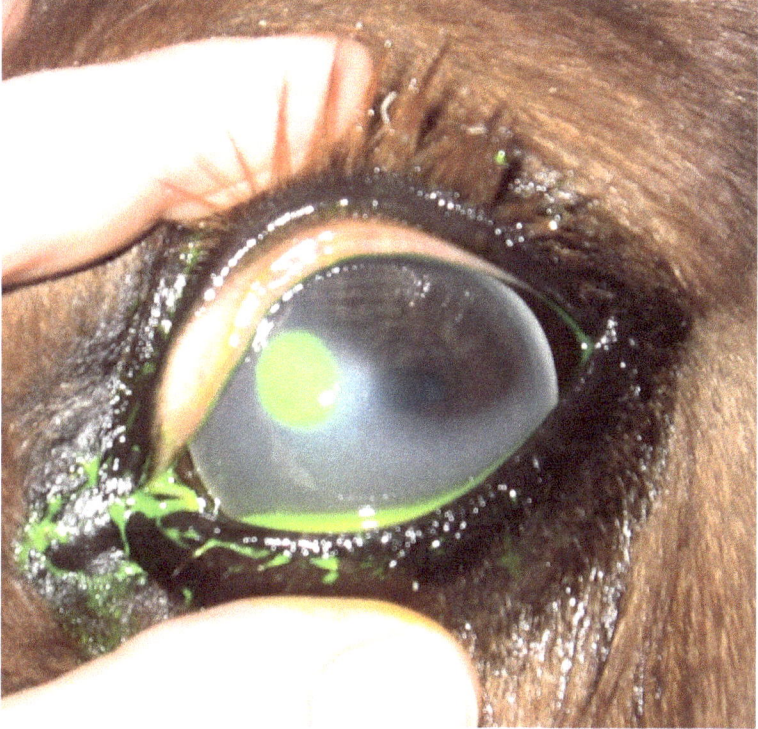

Corneal ulcers are diagnosed with the use of a green stain-fluorescein eye stain.

Ulcers are quite painful.

Seek veterinary care for ulcers because the horse can rub the eye and cause additional injury of the eye or even perforate the cornea easily.

Foreign bodies

Horses are curious animals and are strong. If they encounter danger, they may unintentionally cause an object to injure their eye.

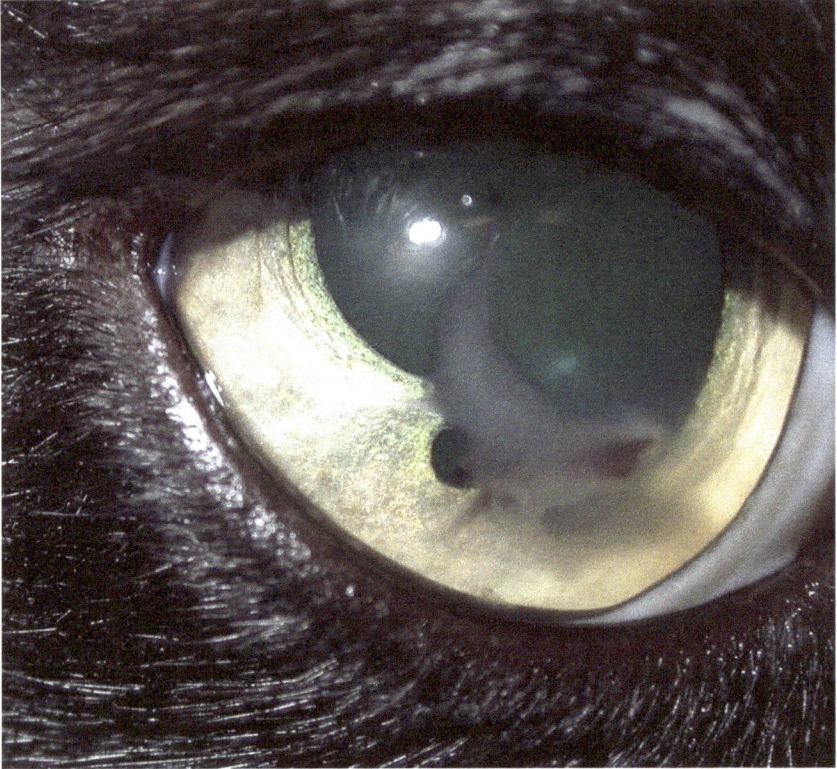

Foreign bodies can be tragic and cause the loss of an eye or loss of vision.

Seek veterinary care immediately for this type of injury.

UVEITIS (MOON BLINDNESS) (ERU)

There are two forms of uveitis. One is fairly treatable and the other is serious and only manageable. This second is known as equine recurrent uveitis.

Equine recurrent uveitis (ERU), also known as moon blindness or periodic ophthalmia, is one of the most common eye conditions in horses and is the leading cause of blindness.

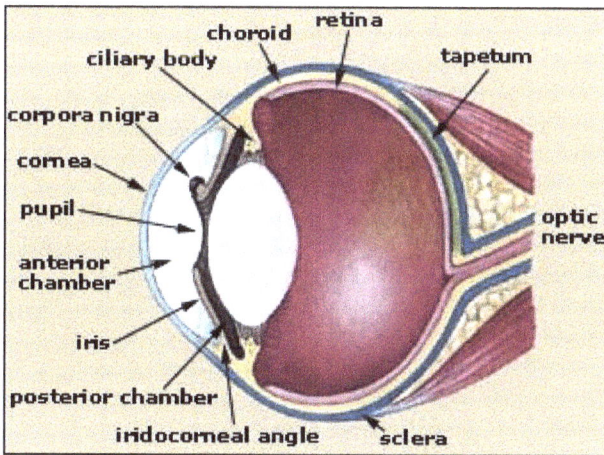

Uveitis- is an irritation/ inflammation in the 'uvea' of the eye. The uvea is the area in the 'middle' structures of the eye that contains the blood vessels- the choroid, ciliary body, and iris (seen above).

ERU is an 'immune-mediated disease- which means the horse's immune system (the system that protects against disease) is abnormally attacking its own tissues in the eye.

The exact cause of the disease is unknown.

There is no cure for ERU.

Appaloosas, paint horses, drafts, and warmbloods seem to be most affected by ERU, while standardbreds and thoroughbreds appear to be less affected

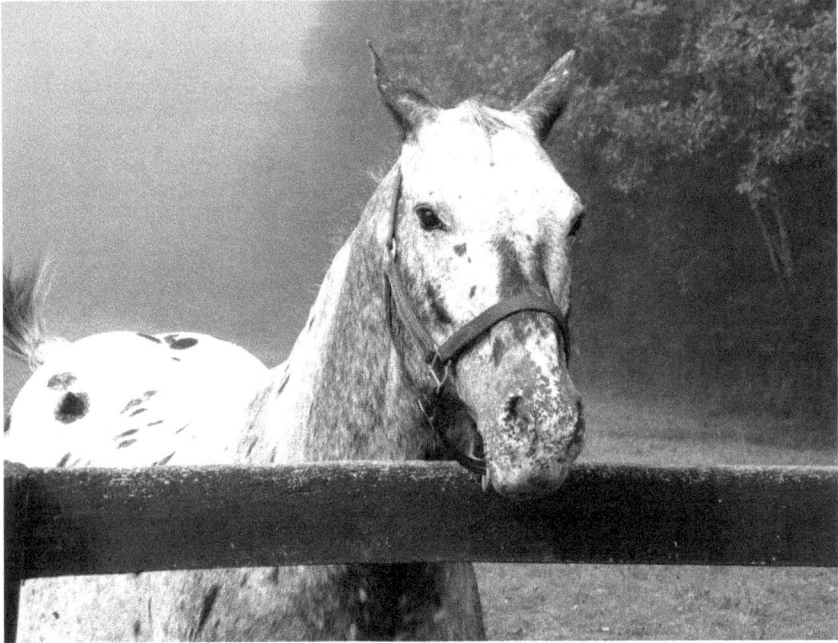

Signs of active uveitis come and go and include:

- sensitivity to light
- squinting
- tearing
- swelling of the cornea- the clear part of the front of the eye
- haziness to the front part of the eye- in front of the iris -that may be bluish
- redness to the eye
- small pupil size
- irregularities to the iris
- loss of vision

Chapter 12

Miscellaneous

How to check a Horse's Temperature, Heart Rate, and Breathing Rate

Checking a Horse's Vital Signs

	Adult	Newborn
Temperature- (use a rectal thermometer)	99-101 °F (37.2-38.3°C)	99.5-102.1 °F (37.5-38.9 °C)
Pulse –	28-55 beats/min	80-100 beats/min

Take the pulse by placing you hand over the chest of the horse or by feeling for an arterial pulse under the jaw x 15 seconds x 4.

Respirations -	10-24 breaths/min	20-40 breaths/min

Take the respiratory rate by watching the chest expand and relax. Count for 15 seconds and x 4.

Common Vital Sign Mistakes

- not leaving the thermometer in long enough – may get low readings if not measured for at least 1 minute
- taking vital signs on a nervous or painful horse - horses' pulse and respiration rates can increase dramatically if they are nervous or in pain
- allowing the horse to sniff a hand to measure respiration rate – the horse will sniff far more quickly than their regular breathing rates
- double-counting heartbeats - lub-dub=one beat
- not regularly checking a horse to know what is normal

EMERGENCIES

Emergencies happen. Being prepared helps during these stressful times.

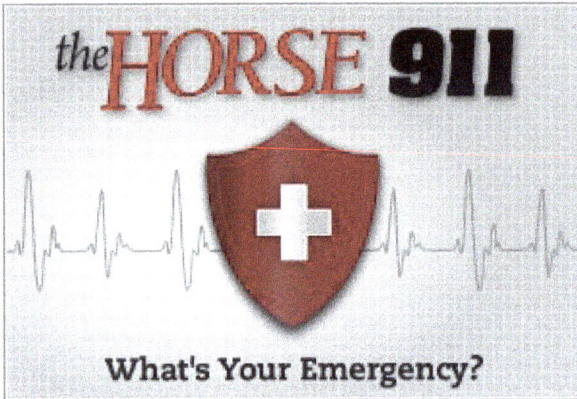

Common horse emergencies include:

- colic
- lacerations (cuts)
- falls
- trailer accidents
- bites
- sudden lameness
- thermal injuries – hot and cold
- eye emergencies
- laminitis
- choke
- broken bones
- poisoning
- snake bite
- reactions to medications or vaccines
- sudden collapse
- lightning strike
- barn fires
- and more

Colic

Colic is a common horse emergency and is a sign, or symptom, of a problem. It is pain in the abdomen of the horse caused by various disorders that causes the signs below seen from the pain.

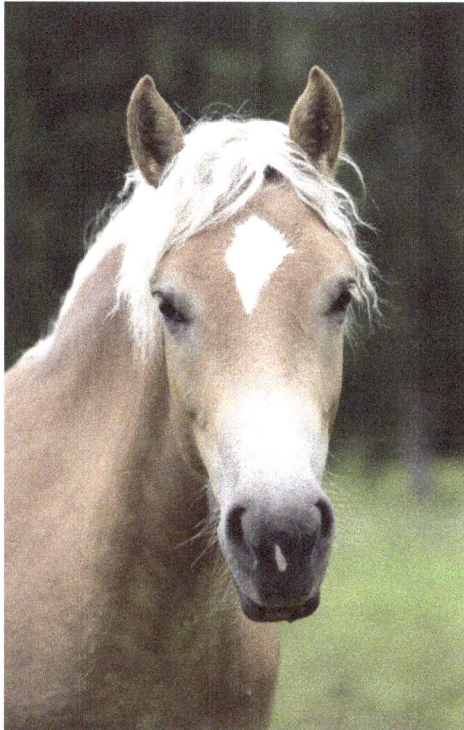

Causes of colic include:

- distention of the intestine with air (gas)
- twisted intestines - a surgical emergency
- impaction of fecal matter
- air (gas) in the stomach – since horses are unable to vomit or eructate (belch, burp), when air distends the stomach it causes pain

Signs of colic include:

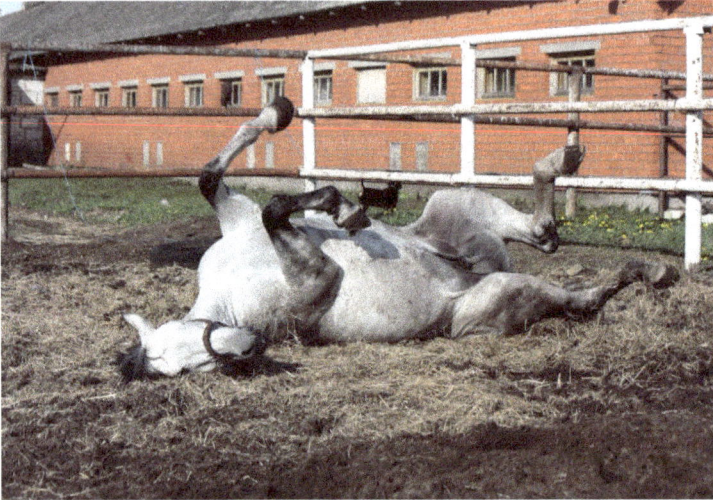

- sweating
- rolling
- kicking
- distention of the abdomen
- high heart rate
- high respiratory rate

Normal intestinal sounds – the normal gut sounds sound like gurgling, growling, and tinkling noises. In colic, abnormal sounds are present- or no sounds of bowel activity.

It is important to keep the horse walking- or off the ground from rolling and contact a veterinarian for care immediately

WHAT TO DO:

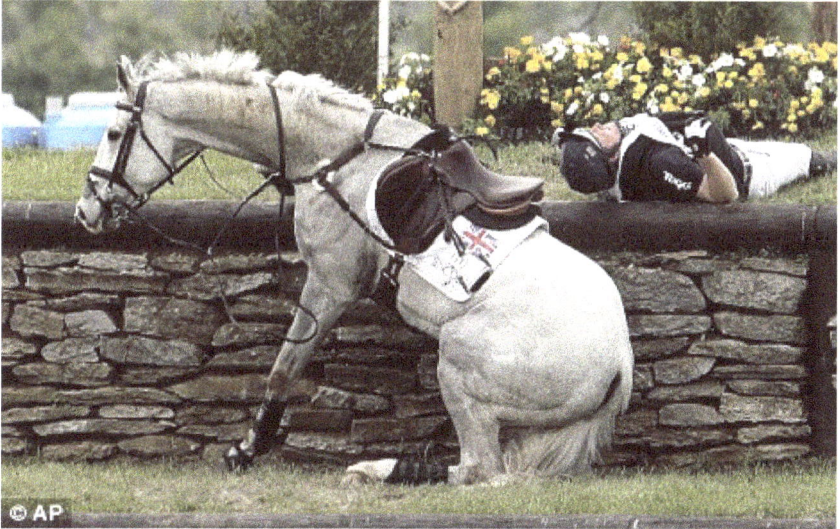

- be prepared - have supplies and know all the emergency clinics' and personal veterinary clinics' phone numbers in the area around the horse's barn/home
- know any dangers in the world around the horse - weather, snakes, plants, animals, and more
- stay with the horse and, if necessary, begin transferring the horse to a veterinary emergency clinic as soon as possible
- while seeking veterinary care, have someone with you if possible

Items to Include in a Home First Aid Kit:

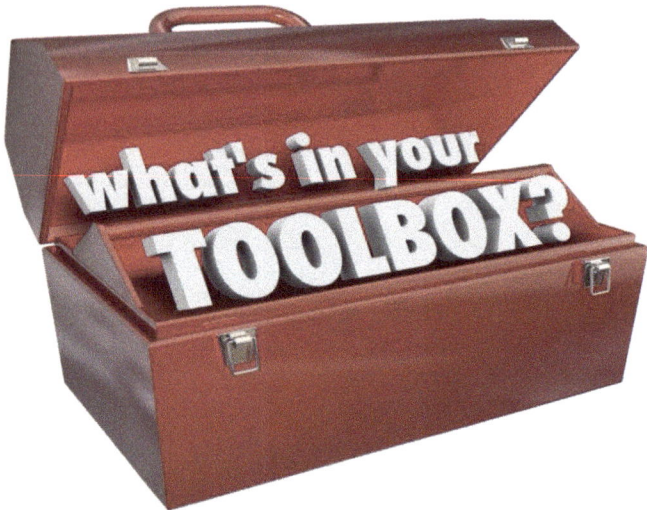

- alcohol (70% isopropyl alcohol-rubbing alcohol)
- antibacterial cream
- bandaging material- gauze pads, gauze rolls, rolls of cotton, self-adhesive wraps such as 'vet wrap' or 'co flex' bandage
- hydrogen peroxide
- rectal thermometer
- scissors
- pliers or nippers to pull nails
- eye wash
- flashlight
- blankets and towels
- tweezers
- the phone numbers to the local emergency clinics
- the phone number to poison control

Keep the kit in a sealed container in your barn.

Examining A Horse

Knowing what a normal exam is for a horse makes it easier to know when veterinary care is needed. It can also help when purchasing a horse. A veterinarian should be consulted for a pre-purchase exam.

Basic Physical Exam is from head to toe -

First- before starting an exam- look at the horse in general- are they awake, active, ears up? happy to see you? moving correctly? How are they standing and breathing? acting normal? in good spirits?

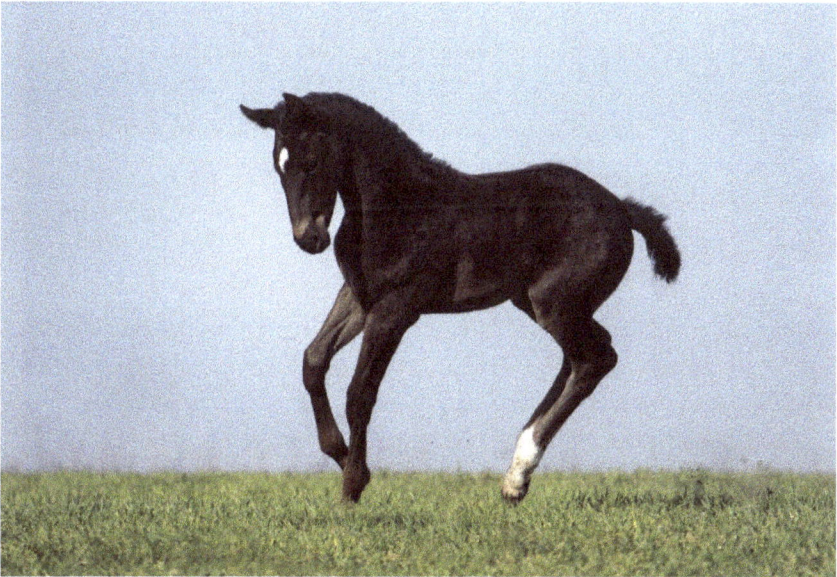

Normal: awake and responsive, responding when called, walking correctly, breathing easily
Not Normal: will not wake up for you, unable to stand, breathing heavily, anything that concerns you

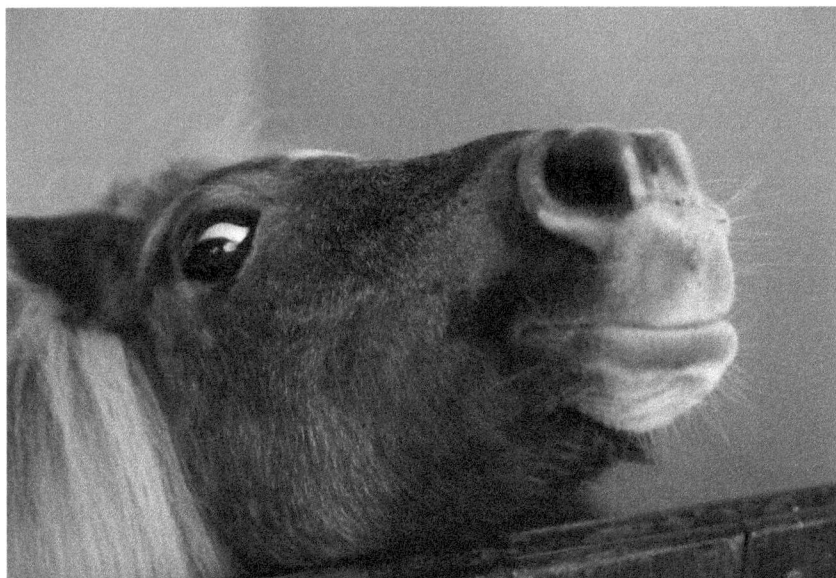

Head: look at the horse's head area

Normal: normal forehead and face, smooth hair coat, no missing hair, no bumps
Not Normal: open wounds, bumps or swelling on surface, the shape of the head not the same on both sides

Eyes: look at both eyes

Normal: bright, moist, clear, equal pupils that are oval shaped, whites of eyes white in color, look the same on both sides, looks at you when you are talking
Not normal: dull, sunken eyes that appear dry or cloudy, colored discharge from the eyes, yellow or red color to the whites of the eyes, squinting, swelling, painful appearance to the eyes, resisting when attempting to open the eyelids, inability to see

(Continued assessment of the head areas)

Ears: look at both ears

Normal: normal hair present if not clipped, no odor, dry, typical carriage of ears, no masses
Not Normal: swelling to any area of the ear, odor, redness, pain, wounds, scabs, rash, not carrying ears the same on both sides- for example- one up, one down, obvious parasites

Nose: look at the nose

Normal: moist and clean
Not Normal: very dry and cracked, colored discharge- white, green, yellow, tan, red, bleeding, swelling, loss of pigment (coloring) of the nose

Throat: look at the throat and gently feel the throat as well

Normal: no cough, no swellings or growths, all areas feel the same on both sides of the neck
Not Normal: cough when gently feeling the neck area, difficulties in breathing, swelling, growths, anything that feels larger on one side than the other

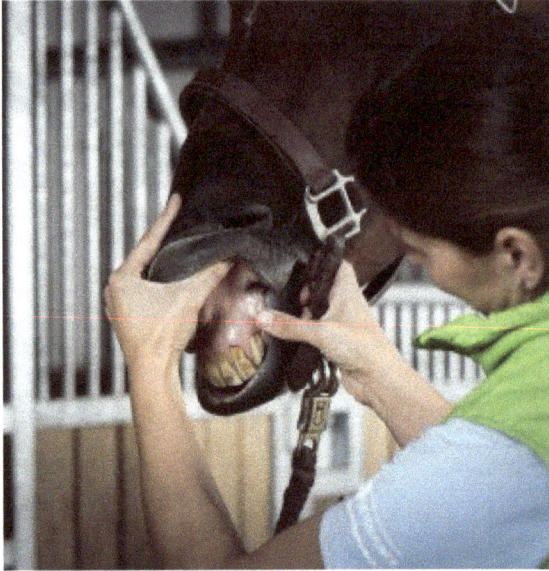

Oral- look at the horse's teeth and open the mouth by turning up the lip fold

Normal: teeth are clean and white, no sharp or uneven edges, the gums are pink
Not Normal: broken teeth, missing teeth, sharp teeth, uneven surfaces of the teeth, reddening of the gums, odor to the mouth or green/tan/yellow discharge from the gums around any teeth, sores in the mouth, growths in the mouth, excess gums over the teeth

MM- the mucous membranes- AKA the gums- look at the area under the lip and above the teeth- what color is it?

Normal: pink
Not Normal: pale pink, cherry red, bluish, yellow

Capillary refill time (CRT) – is completed by lifting the upper lip, pressing the gum above the teeth to make the gum pale and measuring how long it takes to return to pink. 1-2 seconds is normal

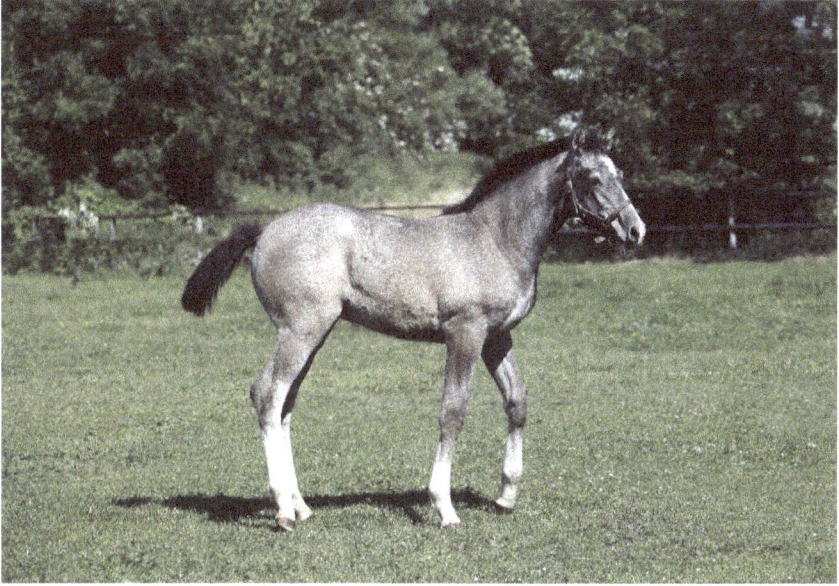

Heart/Lungs- listen for breathing and feel the heart by placing a hand along the side of the horse's chest or placing a hand on the inside of the horse's jaw bone

Normal: regular heart rate and easy breathing, even moving of the chest in and out with breathing

Not Normal: irregular, slow or fast heart rate, any noises heard as the horse breaths, coughing, any visible signs of difficulty breathing- such as opening the mouth to breathe, any blue coloring of the mouth, if the horse is unable to rest or lie down

(Continued assessment of the body areas)

Abdomen- feeling the abdomen of the horse is difficult due to its size, however, you can push on the sides gently pressing into the abdomen – move slowly and gently from the front of the abdomen to the back of the abdomen -it is also possible to listen to the abdomen with a stethoscope

Normal: soft, not painful, slim (if the pet is not overweight), no lumps, bumps, masses, normal rumbling of bowel sounds to every area of the abdomen
Not normal: large, tense, rounded, painful abdomen when touching the horse, any lumps, bumps, or masses, decreased or absent rumbling of bowel sounds in any area of the abdomen

Neurological– exam the pet's ability to walk properly and respond properly

Normal: the horse can feel you touch them; all four feet stand properly on the ground, able to walk in a straight line
Not Normal: head tilting to one side, inability to walk, pain or no pain when pinching areas of the legs, seizures, fainting, inability to wake a pet, hoofs knuckling over

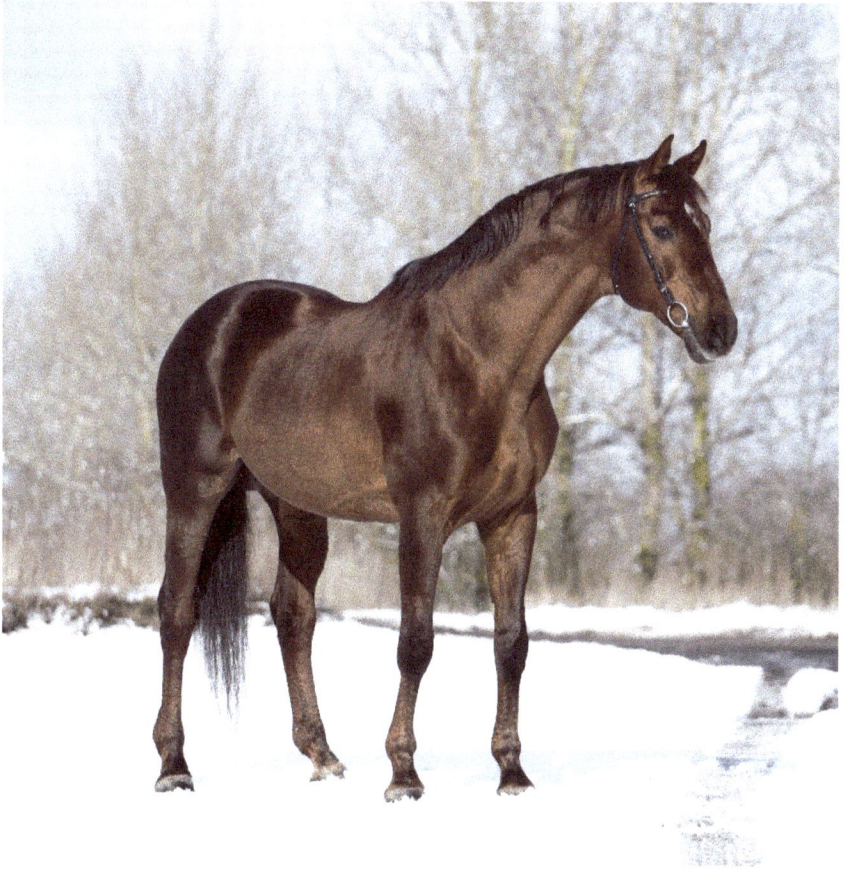

Skin/Coat-look at and feel the pet's skin and hair coat

Normal: shiny, smooth, soft, unbroken hair and smooth skin, minimal odor – only the lovely odor of the horse

Not Normal: sparse or patchy hair coat, open sores or wounds, growths, excess oil in the skin, dry skin, reddening, odor, rash

(Continued assessment of the extremities)

Extremities- look at all 4 legs of the horse

Normal: able to walk evenly on all 4 legs, no deformities, no growths, no swelling
Not Normal: unable to walk on 1 or more legs, swelling, pain when touching areas, growths, dangling legs, open wounds, odor, discharge of any color

Lymph nodes- these may be difficult to locate on a horse unless they are enlarged

Normal: unable to feel lymph nodes
Not Normal: swelling in the areas of the lymph nodes- under the jaw, in front of the front legs, in front of the back legs, behind the knees, in the groin or under the front legs

Muscles and bones- look at the horse's back and legs and muscles over the body

Normal: muscles soft and covering the bones evenly on both sides of the body part being examined, able to walk without pain
Not Normal: small muscle size in any area, tense muscles, pain when gently feeling over the spine and other body areas, pain when walking, jumping, or playing

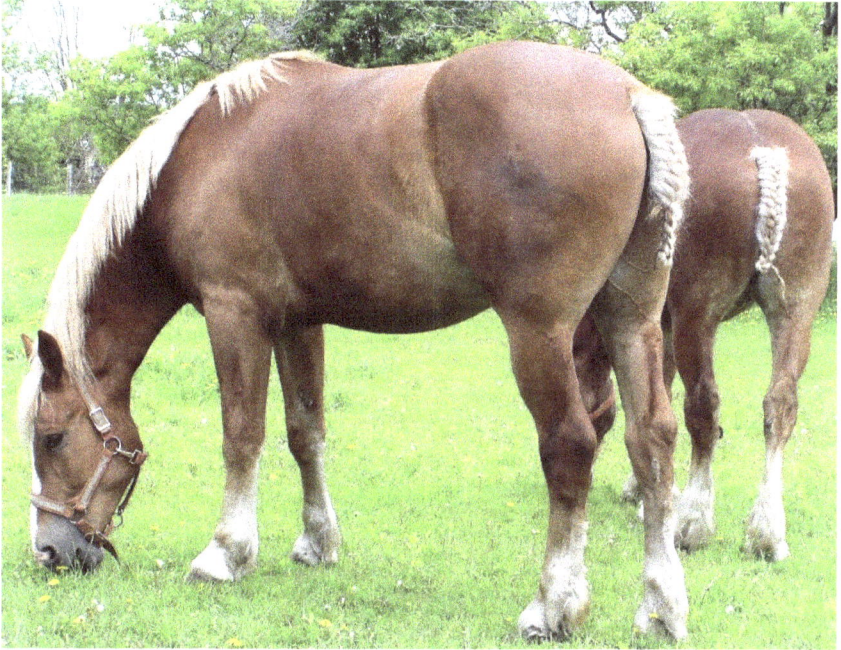

Urogenital- exam the horse's ability to pass urine and the male and female parts of the horse

Normal: clean and dry areas- no discharge, swelling, pain
Not Normal: any swelling, discharge, odor, inability to urinate

Perineum- examine the area under the tail area

Normal: clean and dry, no swelling
Not Normal: swelling, discharge, odor, masses

Tail– examine the pet's tail

Normal: able to hold tail up, able to move the tail
Not Normal: inability to move tail, growths, swelling, pain, crooked tail, open wounds

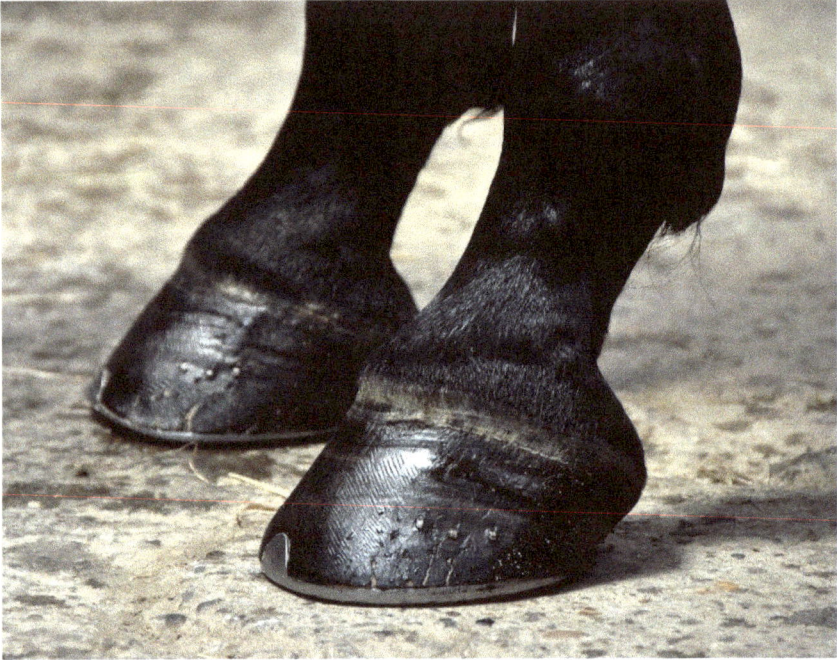

Feet – examine the horse's feet and hooves

Normal: hooves are an appropriate length and clean and dry, no irregularities to any areas of the feet/hooves, warm to the touch
Not Normal: swelling in any area of the hoof, discharge from any area of the hoof, thick, discolored, misshapen hooves, curvature of the hooves upward or downward

Senior Horses

Caring for the Older Horse

Good nutrition, maintenance, and veterinary care have allowed horses to lead longer and more productive lives- even into their late 20s and 30s.

However, as the horse ages, its needs change, and additional care may be required to keep the horse as healthy as possible.

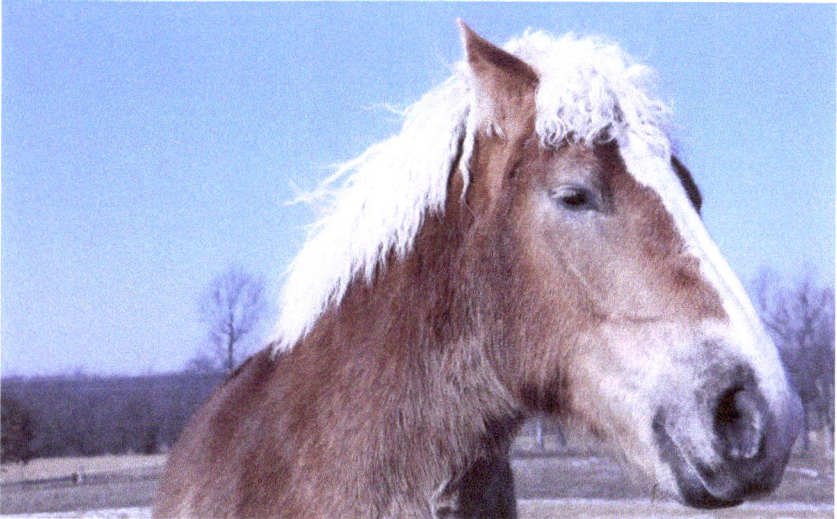

Key areas to consider when caring for the older horse are:

- nutrition
- dentition
- lameness
- vision
- immune system changes
- hormonal changes

261

Nutrition/ Dentition

Some older horses may not have teeth or may have missing, abscessed, or unevenly worn teeth as mentioned in chapter 6.

This problem may easily be solved by changing the type of food the older horse eats.

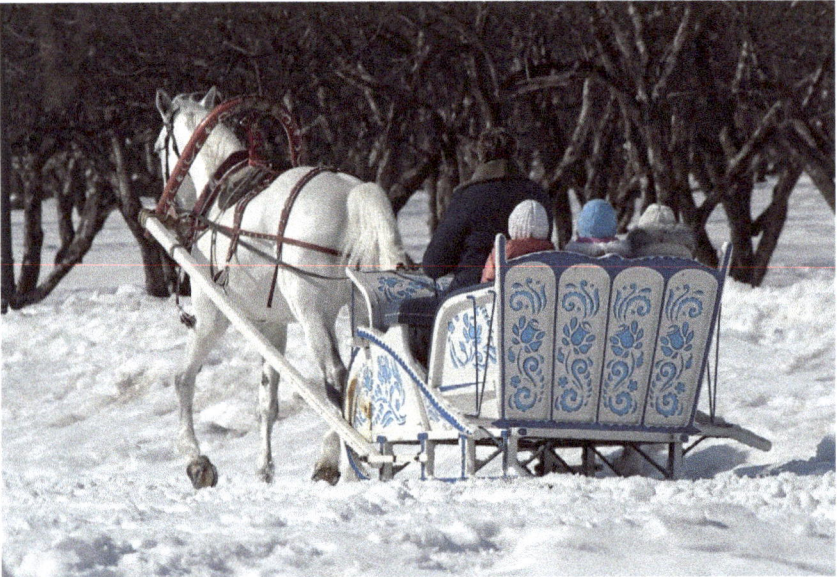

Forage can be provided in the form of hay cubes or pellets (made of either alfalfa or alfalfa/grass mix), which can also be wet down and softened for the horse to chew easily.

Feed companies make senior horse feeds that are softer in texture and some are in the form of pellets.

These pelleted feeds can be wet down and softened even more to make a gruel that is easy for the horse to chew. Also, the horse only needs to swallow the pellets to obtain nutrition. Chewing is not mandatory for receiving nutrients.

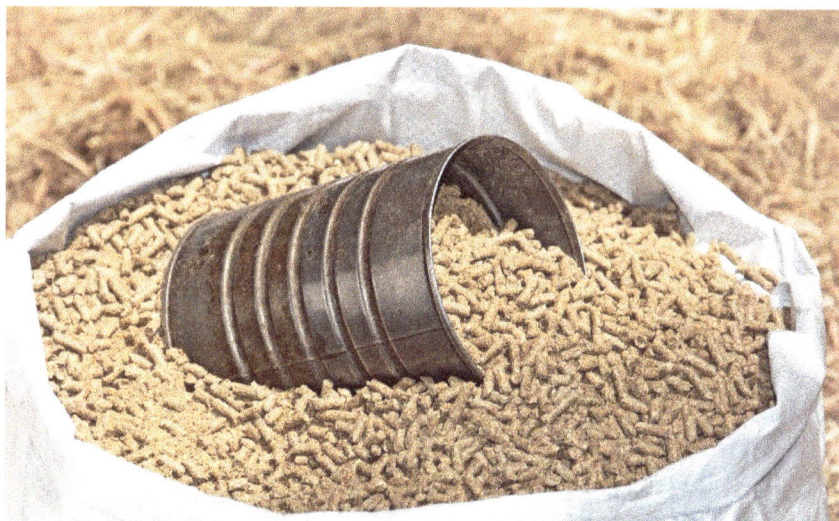

Remember not to overfeed. Older horses may be less active. Excess weight is difficult on joints and whole body areas of senior horses.

Water is critical. Sometimes warming the water- especially in colder climates/seasons helps increase water intake.

In Conclusion

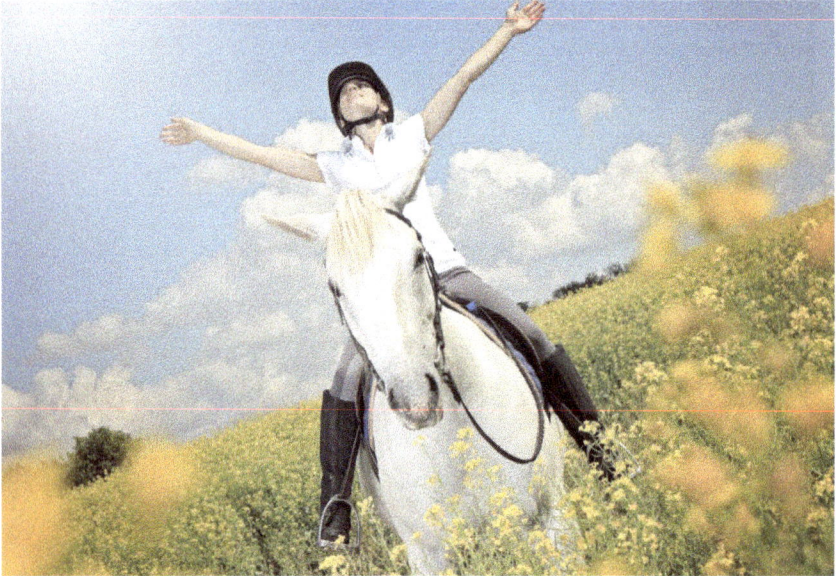

Ex – hil – a – rate – A verb – to make cheerful or merry, enliven, invigorate, stimulate.

Horses are exhilarating!

Whether you just want to go….

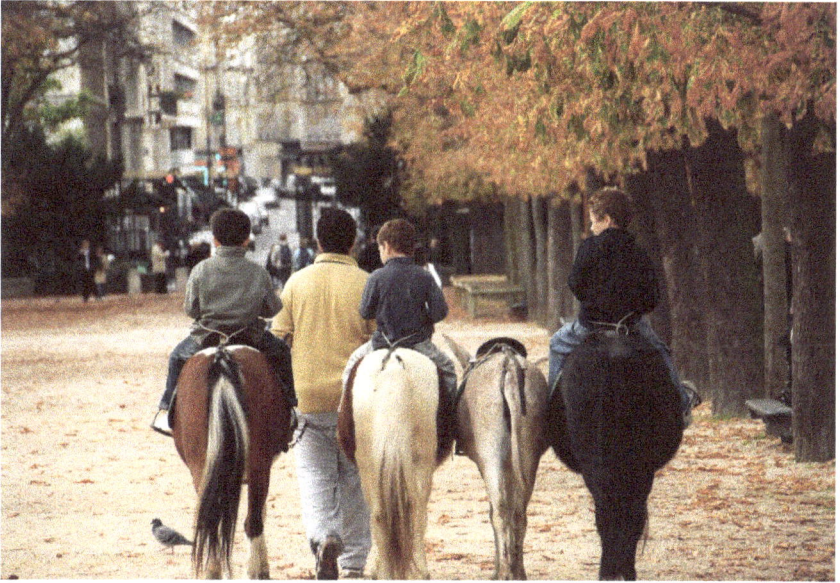

`

….for a leisurely ride….

.......are just trying to have some time…

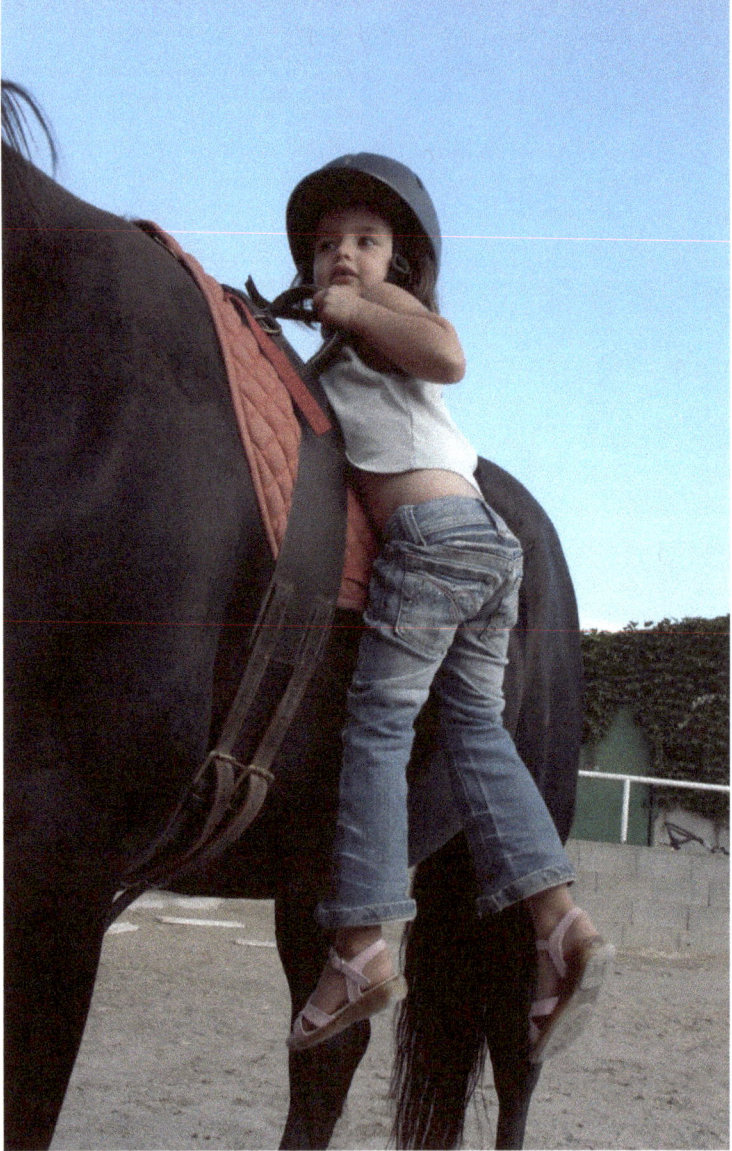

….in the saddle……

….have a few cattle…

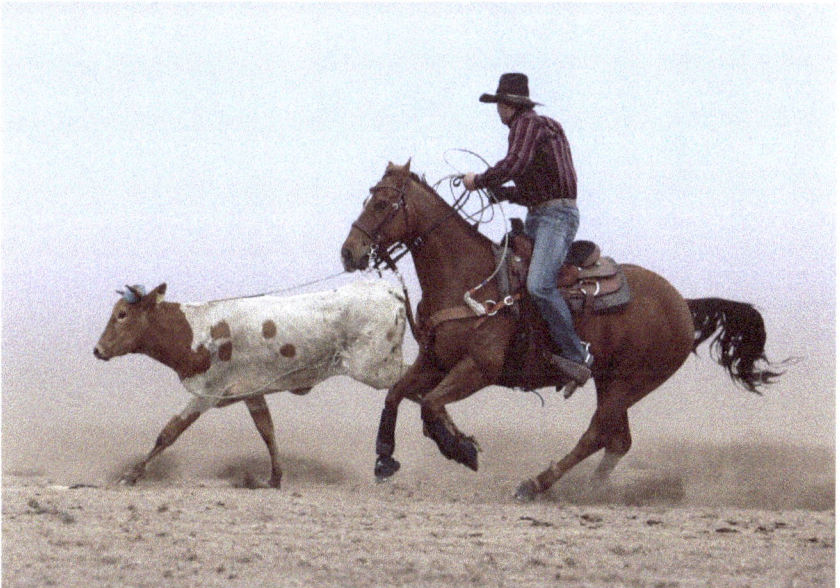

.....to cut……

.… want to train….

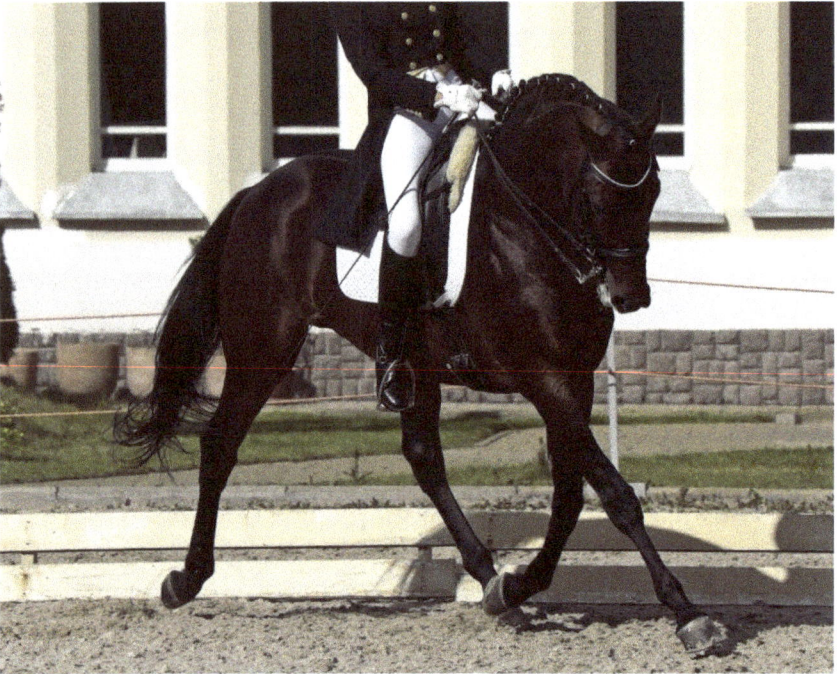

…..an elegant horse…..

......have a show ...

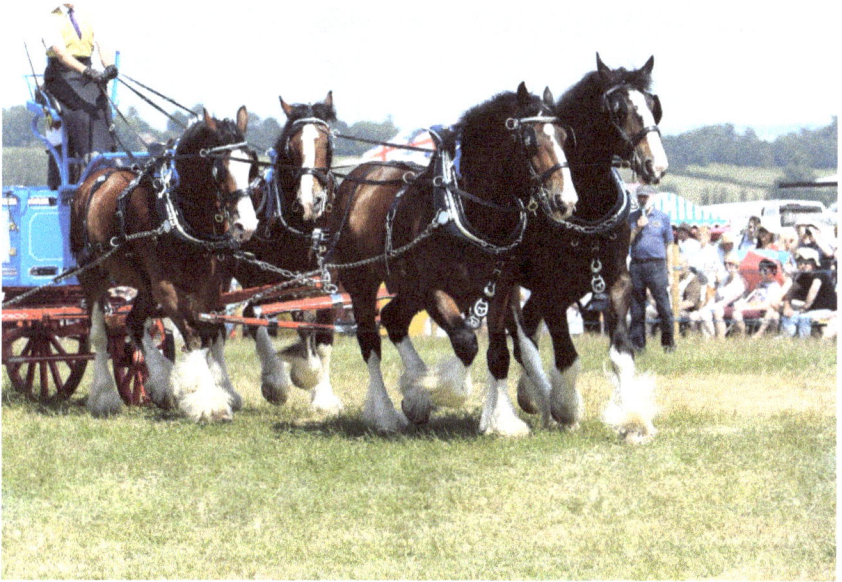

....to put on....

... or enjoy….

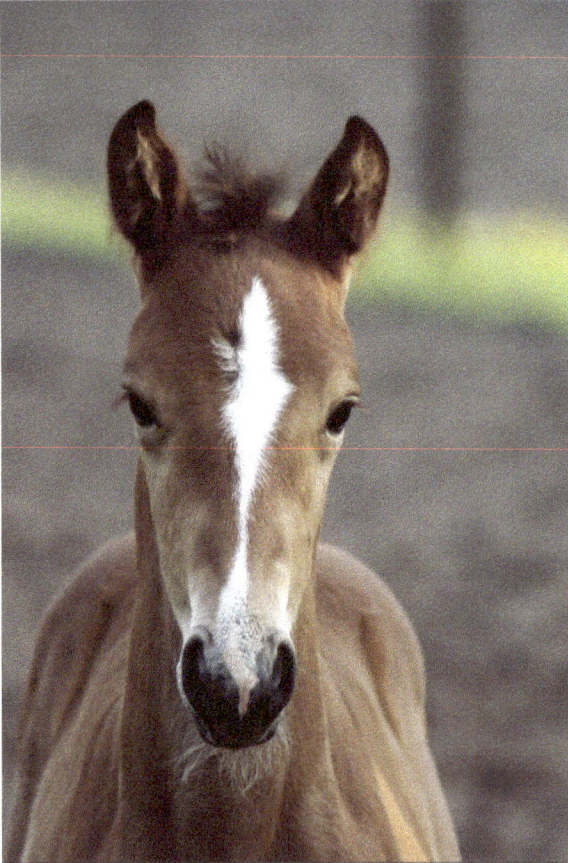

…raising baby horses…..

All horse owners have one thing in common….

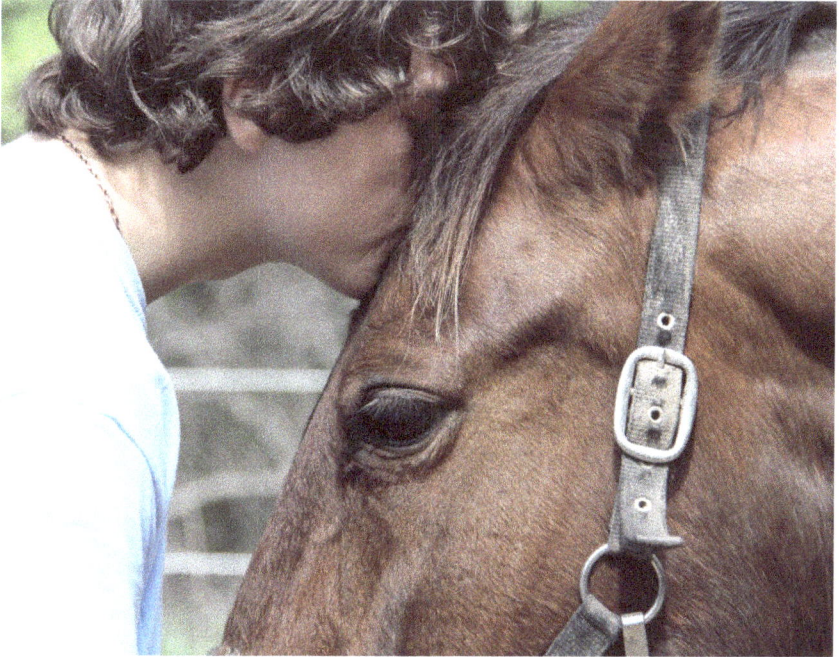

….they love their horses!